LABORATORY MANUAL OF
HISTOLOGY

GEORGE S. PAPPAS
IONA COLLEGE
NEW ROCHELLE, NEW YORK

 Wm. C. Brown Publishers

Book Team

Editor *Edward G. Jaffe*
Developmental Editor *Janette S. Stecki*
Production Coordinator *Kay Driscoll*

WCB **Wm. C. Brown Publishers**

President *G. Franklin Lewis*
Vice President, Editor-in-Chief *George Wm. Bergquist*
Vice President, Director of Production *Beverly Kolz*
Vice President, National Sales Manager *Bob McLaughlin*
Director of Marketing *Thomas E. Doran*
Advertising Manager *Ann M. Knepper*
Marketing Manager *Craig S. Marty*
Executive Editor *Edward G. Jaffe*
Production Editorial Manager *Colleen A. Yonda*
Production Editorial Manager *Julie A. Kennedy*
Publishing Services Manager *Karen J. Slaght*
Manager of Visuals and Design *Faye M. Schilling*

Cover photo © Edwin Reschke

Copyright © 1990 by Wm. C. Brown Publishers. All rights reserved

Library of Congress Catalog Card Number: 89–60283

ISBN 0–697–09715–3

No part of this publication may be reproduced, stored in a retrieval
system, or transmitted, in any form or by any means, electronic,
mechanical, photocopying, recording, or otherwise, without the
prior written permission of the publisher.

Printed in the United States of America by Wm. C. Brown Publishers,
2460 Kerper Boulevard, Dubuque, IA 52001

10 9 8 7 6 5 4 3 2 1

Contents

Preface

Most courses in histology are taught in conjunction with a standard textbook and atlas. For the typical laboratory, however, there are few, if any, major published laboratory guides that lead the student through the pedagogic steps of basic review, observation of histologic material, drawings, and the answering of questions. This manual provides, in addition, an optional exercise in histological technique. To answer the questions at the end of each chapter, the student will need to research the answers in standard texts and other reference sources. The material is presented in 15 chapters, which coincides with the typical length of a college semester of 15 weeks of study. Although the primary audience for this manual is the upper level undergraduate student of histology, the manual may be used by any level prehealth professions student and also by students in professional school.

At the end of each chapter are student exercises. The student is expected to label prepared illustrations with terms listed. Slide lists and labels are also provided. After microscopic examination of the slides, the student is expected to make original drawings in the spaces provided and to identify structures using the labels provided as a guide. Although many excellent texts and atlases are available, most of which supply numerous illustrations from light and electron microscopy, few students in courses of histology are afforded the opportunity or time for a hands-on experience with both the light and electron microscope. Therefore, this manual will present realistically study material that relates mostly to the light microscopic anatomy of tissues and will only make textual reference to electron microscopy.

I wish to acknowledge Dr. Warren Rosenberg of Iona College for his editorial review and valuable suggestions and for providing the electron micrographs. In addition, I wish to thank Dr. Joseph F. Gennaro of New York University for editorial suggestions, Patricia A. Gast for line drawings, Lucy Perazzo for typing and editorial assistance, Luigi Albano for preparation of the index, and my wife, Margaret, for her patience and encouragement.

Drawings

"Whoever does not draw, does not observe."
Leonardo da Vinci

Artistic ability is not required to make careful drawings of structures you observe under the microscope. Simple line drawings are powerful self-teaching aids that will help you to learn and remember the essential structural relationships of cells and tissues.

Begin by drawing an outline of the microscope field section. Then select areas of special interest or a representative area and complete it in detail showing particular structures or cellular organization including expanded scale if necessary. All significant structures must be labeled in print.

Suggestions:

1. Draw a small area at a time, referring constantly to the slide under the microscope and to related textbook and laboratory manual descriptions.
2. Note the form, size, and organization of the area in relation to other areas in the field.
3. It is better to draw the object large rather than small.
4. Use a sharp, hard pencil to make your drawings first; then you may color the structures to correspond with the color of the stain. If known, indicate the stain used by printing next to the title.
5. Always bring your textbook to the laboratory session to aid in identifying objects and to provide a description of the material under study.

Chapter 1

The Cell

Introduction to Cells and Tissues

The vital functional biological units of living matter are the *cells,* a term coined by Robert Hooke in 1665 when he observed microscopic sections of cork tissue. However, it was not until 1838 that Matthias Schleiden, an erratic, volatile lawyer who had turned to biology, and Theodore Schwann, a German physiologist, developed the cell theory. The theory, briefly stated, maintains that "all living things are composed of cells and cell products." The next major advance was the pronouncement in 1858 by noted German pathologist, Rudolf Virchow, that "cells arise from preexisting cells." This was followed in 1861 with the noted histological researches of Max Schultz, who proposed that the basic gelatinouslike substance of plant and animal cells was a material called *protoplasm,* a term first used by Jan Purkinje in 1839 and is the "physical basis of life" as stated by T. Huxley in 1868.

The basic biological unit that has properties associated with life is the *cell.* The average size of a cell is approximately 15 micrometers (μ). Although many components of living cells may be identified, these subcellular units, or organelles, such as mitochondria and Golgi are not in themselves living units even though they may be integral parts of a cell.

Although cells are the ultimate building blocks of the body, these cells are organized into a higher level of complexity in the formation of *tissues.* The English word tissue is taken from the French *tissu* (weave or texture) referring to a cloth or fabric, which in turn is derived from the Greek *istos* meaning tissue or web. This concept was introduced by M. F. X. Bichat, an eighteenth century French anatomist, who, after having performed many dissections observed the different layers, structures, and textures of the body. These observations were made without the use of a microscope and he subsequently wrote a book describing the tissues of the body classifying more than 20 varieties.

His work was continued by others and the special study of the minute structure of the tissues came to be called *histology.* This term, introduced by Richard Owen in 1844, is derived from a Greek word meaning "something woven."

With the subsequent improvement of microscopy, four basic types of tissues were accepted by biologists—although these basic types include various subtypes. The four basic types of tissue are (1) epithelial, (2) connective (loose connective tissue, e.g., fat, blood, and lymph, and dense connective tissue, e.g., bone, tendon, and ligament), (3) nervous, and (4) muscle. The science of histology deals with the microscopic and ultramicroscopic anatomy of the fundamental cells, tissues, and organs of the body, and in its broader aspect, correlates structural features with function.

Living organisms, or systems, after millions of years of biological evolution have developed specific structural organization that falls within certain limits.

In evolution, the early unicellular forms evolved, for a variety of reasons, into multicellular forms. This was obviously of survival value as we can readily observe in the world about us. The need to evolve into multicellularity was based on the problems of limited cellular diffusion and transport of nutrients and metabolites. The result was a maximum limit on cell size followed by many cells working in cooperation with one another, which in due course led to specialization of labor and to specialization of cells.

Daniel Mazia, in his 1961 classic work "The Cell," stated,

> The dimensions of cells are, in a rough way quite uniform, no true cells falling below 1 micrometer and few being larger than 1 millimeter in average diameter. The upper limits are probably smaller than this if we exclude cells containing large amounts of storage material and if we restrict ourselves to those having diploid nuclear equipment. It is unlikely that this state of affairs represents a divine dispensation in favor of the manufacturers of microscopes, but it is highly probable that the limits of efficient cell diameter are set by the rates of diffusion of metabolites. By and large, organisms have solved their diffusion problems by producing small cells with single diploid nuclei, providing a large ratio of cell surface to volume.

Cells of multicellular organisms, in meeting the demands of specialization of labor, have evolved many structural features to accommodate various functional needs. Egg cells are relatively large in order to accommodate supplies of yolk; sperm cells are small since they are composed mostly of nuclear material and are motile; nerve cells are elongate because of their axons, which are needed to connect other neural components; and fat cells are usually large because of stored lipids.

The light microscope is still the most common type of microscope used in basic histology. It must be noted, however, that in advanced and research situations, other types of microscopes are used such as the phase-contrast microscope used especially for living cells; the dark-field microscope, which uses a special condenser for producing a dark field enhancing contrast; microscopes that utilize ultraviolet rays, x-rays, and polarized light for observing specimens and enhancing resolution, density, or birefringence. In a transmission electron microscope (EM), a beam of electrons is accelerated to a high velocity in a vacuum. The electron beam is projected through a specimen and focused on a fluorescent screen or photographic plate by means of electromagnetic fields that serve as lenses. The optimum resolution possible with the light microscope is approximately 0.5 μm whereas the electron microscope can resolve cell structures as small as 0.5 nanometers (nm). In the scanning electron microscope (SEM), the electron beam scans the coated surface of a specimen. Reflected electrons are converted into electrical signals that are viewed on a television screen. The resulting three-dimensional image reveals surface contours of the specimen.

The advent of electron microscopy necessitates an alteration of the older terminology used as units of measurement of cells and especially of small ultracellular fine structures. The current system relates more closely to the metric system as follows:

Previous terminology		Current terminology
Micron (μ) or 0.001 mm	=	Micrometer (μm)
Millimicron (mμ) or 0.001μ	=	Nanometer (nm)
Angstrom unit (Å) or 0.1 m	=	0.1 nm

Cell Components and Cell Diversity

In the organization of living matter, cells are considered as the basic living biological unit. Specialized cells are organized into specialized tissues resulting in diverse and efficient additional organizational units, the organs, organ systems, and subsequently the entire organism. These biological units function in an altruistic manner that is essential to the well-being and survival of the organism as a complete unit.

Below the cellular level, however, we have cell components and organelles that do not function as living units independent of the cell. Examples of these cell components and organelles are the cell membrane, the nucleus and its components, and the cytoplasm and cytoplasmic organelles.

The *cell membrane* (plasma membrane or plasmalemma) is a 7–11 nm-thick limiting membrane that encloses the cell and its contents. Because of its small diameter, it typically is not observed under the light microscope unless special staining techniques are used or oblique sections are employed. The cell membrane serves as a selective barrier regulating the transport of materials into and out of the cell. The well-known Danielli-Davson model for the plasma membrane proposes a lipid center with a coat of protein on each surface. In this trilaminar structure, the central lipid bilayer is composed of phospholipids, glycolipids, and cholesterol with their nonpolar or hydrophobic portions in the central core and the polar hydrophilic parts facing the outer sides. More recent evidence (Singer-Nicholson) suggests that the membrane proteins are not continuous but may drift within the lipid bilayer and are arranged either as transmembrane proteins (integral or intrinsic-type) or as peripheral proteins (extrinsic-type). The cell membrane is also characterized by having an external coating of a carbohydrate-containing material known as the cell coat, or glycocalyx.

A *nucleus* is found in all eukaryote cells except mature mammalian erythrocytes. Nuclear shape may be spherical, ovoid, indented, or lobulated. Nuclear size will normally range from 3 to 14 μm in diameter. Cells may be binucleate such as some cardiac muscle cells or parenchymal liver cells. Osteoclasts and skeletal muscle cells may be multinucleate. Cells lacking a nucleus such as mature erythrocytes are incapable of protein synthesis, cannot undergo cell division, and, as a result, have a limited life span. The nucleus in eukaryote cells is bound by a porous 40 nm double nuclear envelope composed of two 7 nm membranes enclosing a 25 nm space. The nuclear membrane pores range 40–100 nm in diameter and are involved in nucleo-cytoplasmic transport. Within the nucleus is the colloidal, semifluid karyoplasm (nuclear sap) in which is suspended the chromatin and the nucleolus. The nuclear chromatin is composed of nucleoproteins, which in turn are composed of proteins, primarily histamines, and DNA (deoxyribonucleic acid) plus RNA (ribonucleic acid). The chromatin is basophilic, is typically stained by hematoxylin stains, and is Feulgen positive (Schiff reaction). Long, thin chromatin threads forming a network of diffuse, thin nucleoprotein threads that represent potentially active regions on DNA strands where transcription can take place are called euchromatin. Condensed regions representing additional quantities of coiled chromatin reflecting inactive DNA and suggesting reduced transcription are referred to as heterochromatin. Heterochromatin is markedly stained by basic dyes and is increasingly evident near the end of the cell's life. During cell division, the chromatin threads become condensed into chromosomes (figs. 1.1, 1.2).

The apparently clear substance within the nucleus is the *karyoplasm,* or *nuclear sap,* in which the nucleolus and chromatin appear suspended. The karyoplasm is a colloidal suspension containing some granules, protein, and dispersed

Figure 1.1 Electron micrograph of liver hepatocyte illustrating typical cell organelles: NuEn = nuclear envelope; NuPo = nuclear pore; EuCh = euchromatin; HCh = heterochromatin; M = mitochondria; Cr = cristae; Gr = mitochondrial granules; V = cytoplasmic vesicle; L = lysosome. (x 53,000).

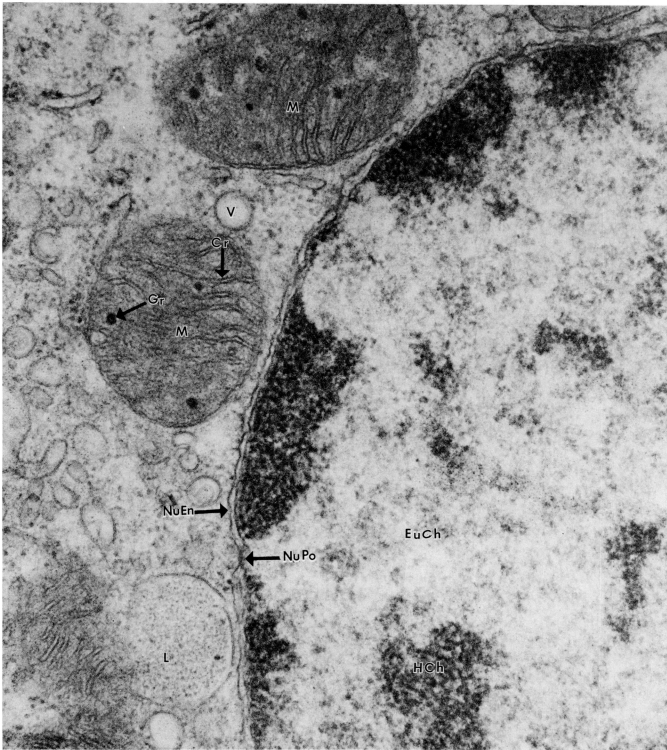

Liver Hepatocyte

NuE—nuclear envelope   Cr—Cristae
NuPo—nuclear pore   Gr—Mitochandral graucles
EuCh—Euchrourotin   V—Chyoplaswic vesicle
Hch—Heterochromatiu   L—Lysosome
M—Mituchondria

Figure 1.2 Electron micrograph of nuclear envelope and nuclear pores: NuEn = nuclear envelope; NuPo = nuclear pore; Ka = karyoplasm; EuCh = euchromatin; HCh = heterochromatin; RNP = ribonucleoprotein particles. (x 160,000).

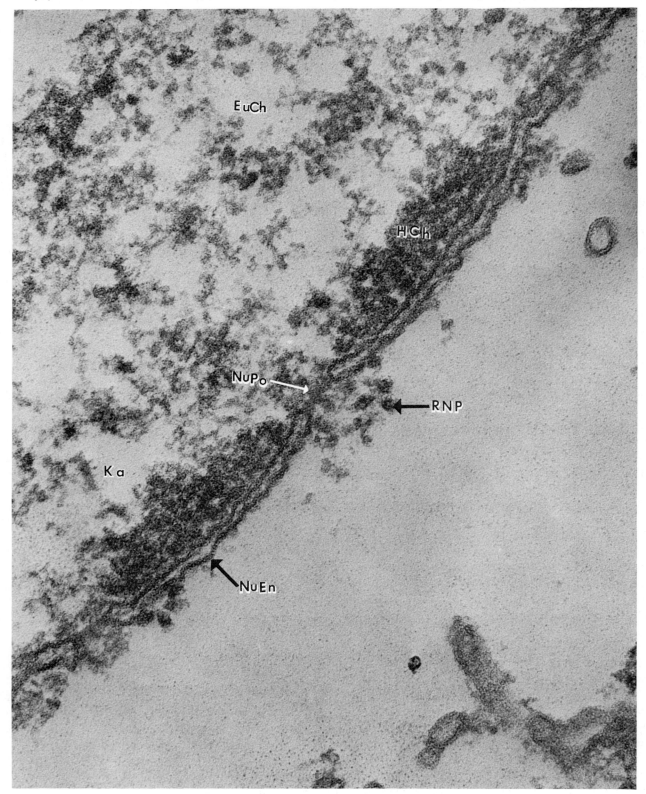

Nuclear Envelop and Pores

NuEn—nuclear envelop	Euch—Euchromatin
NuPo—nuclear pore	Hch—Heterochromatin
Ka—karyoplasm	RNP—Ribonvdeo protein Particles

chromatin. It functions as a medium for the diffusion of metabolites and macromolecules. The *nucleolus* is a non-membrane-bound spherical or ovoid body about 1 μm in diameter and lying within the karyoplasm. It consists of rRNA and molecules, which combine with it to form ribosomes. The nucleolus contains a small amount of DNA. The number and size of nucleoli is constant for particular cell types, however, the interphase nucleus exhibits one to four nucleoli. The nucleoli disappear in late mitotic prophase and reappear during the telophase stage. Nucleoli are usually basophilic due to the RNA content and are typically Feulgen negative. Nucleoli lie on specific sites on chromosomes called nucleolar organizing sites where ribosomal transcription takes place. Consequently, nucleoli are prominent in cells actively engaged in protein synthesis.

Cell organelles include centrioles, cilia and flagella, microtubules and microfilaments. Cytoplasmic organelles typically include ribosomes, endoplasmic reticulum, Golgi apparatus, lysosomes, and mitochondria.

Centrioles appear in light microscopy as two granules, cylinders, or rods near the nucleus or nuclear indentation. They most often appear near the center of the cell thus giving rise to their name. As cylinders or rods they are arranged at right angles to each other and lie in a specialized cytoplasmic area called the centrosome. Their size is 0.5 μm in length and 0.2 μm in diameter. The walls of the cylinders are composed of nine triplets of microtubules embedded in a fine, fibrillar material, the axial component, appearing as a central hub with nine radiating spokes. The microtubules contain the protein tubulin. Centrioles are important in mitosis and function as microtubule organizing centers.

Cilia and *flagella* are hairlike motile structures extending from the cell surface. Cilia range in size from about 0.2 μm in diameter and up to 10 μm in length. Cilia are found on the surface of epithelial cells of the upper respiratory tract, in parts of the male and female reproductive tract, and on the ependymal cells lining the central nervous system. The same fundamental ultrastructural arrangement is seen in the cilia of all animal cells. The surface of a ciliated cell may contain up to 250 or more cilia.

Electron microscopy reveals an internal structure of two central microtubules and nine peripheral pairs of fused double microtubules or doublets. This arrangement of microtubules is called the *axoneme*. Cilia are covered by an extension of the plasmalemma. A *basal body* is seen as a dense granule at the base of the cilium. The basal body exhibits an ultrastructure identical to that of centrioles. In the development of cilia, centrioles replicate to provide a basal body that, in turn, is involved in microtubule generation resulting in cilia formation. Flagella have the same basic ultrastructure as cilia but are longer by ranging up to 70 μm in length. They are usually present as but one or two per cell and are typically seen in the tail of mammalian spermatozoan and as vestigial structures of uncertain function in the epithelium of the collecting duct of the kidney tubule.

Ribosomes are electron dense, roughly spherical, cytoplasmic particles 15–25 nm in diameter. Ribosomes contain RNA and protein, are responsible for cytoplasmic basophilia, and are prevalent in protein synthesizing cells such as pancreatic and salivary acinar cells and also lymphoblasts, myeloblasts, and osteoblasts. These particles are sites of protein synthesis where amino acids are incorporated into peptides resulting in specific protein formation. Ribosomes may be attached to the outer nuclear membrane and typically to the endoplasmic reticulum.

The *endoplasmic reticulum* (ER) is composed of a series of tubules and broad, flattened membranous sacs, the cisternae, which are arranged in interconnecting sheets. The ER that is associated with ribosomes is termed rough or granular endoplasmic reticulum (rER). The membrane of the ER has a unit structure 6–7 nm thick enclosing a lumen or intracisternal space of 50 nm. This space contains newly synthesized protein, which is transported within the ER to the Golgi region where it is concentrated. The ER that is not lined with ribosomes is called smooth-surfaced (agranular) endoplasmic reticulum (sER). The sER is more tubular and vesicular rather than cisternal. The size of the membranes and tubular lumen of sER is similar to that of rER. The sER is well represented in steroid secreting cells such as the Leydig cells of the testis, which secrete testosterone; the adrenocortical cells, which secrete corticosteroids; the corpus luteum of the ovary where progesterone is secreted; liver parenchymal cells involved in the conversion of glycogen to glucose; and intestinal epithelial cells associated with lipid absorption (fig. 1.3).

The *Golgi apparatus,* Golgi complex, or simply Golgi is a network of canals or closely packed laminar membranous cisternae associated with vacuoles or vesicles, lacking ribosomes, and typically located near the cell nucleus. This organelle was first identified by the neurologist Camillo Golgi in 1898 using silver salt impregnation techniques. Golgi, along with another eminent neurologist, Santiago Ramon y Cajal, shared the Nobel prize in 1906 for their work on nerve cells. Although the existence of this organelle was not firmly established until the advent of the electron microscope, it is now well established that the Golgi is involved in concentrating, packaging, and sorting secretory products of cells. The cisternae are arranged in parallel stacks of 3 to 12, with a spacing of 20 to 30 nm between adjacent cisternae. The cisternae may show pores and tubular expansions on the peripheral surfaces. The membrane of the cisternae is 6 to 7 nm wide on the inner forming surface, and 7.5–10 nm wide on the outer surface. The lumen of the cisternae will average about 15 nm. The Golgi is prevalent in secretory cells such as the acinar cells of the pancreas, which secrete pancreatic enzymes; in goblet cells of intestinal epithelium, which secret sulfated mucopolysaccharides; and in the beta cells of the pancreas, which secret insulin (figs. 1.3, and 1.4).

Figure 1.3 Secretory organelles from pancreatic acinar cell: Go = Golgi; RER = rough endoplasmic reticulum; V = secretory vesicle; R = ribosomal particle; Lu = er lumen; M = mitochondrion; Col = collagaen.

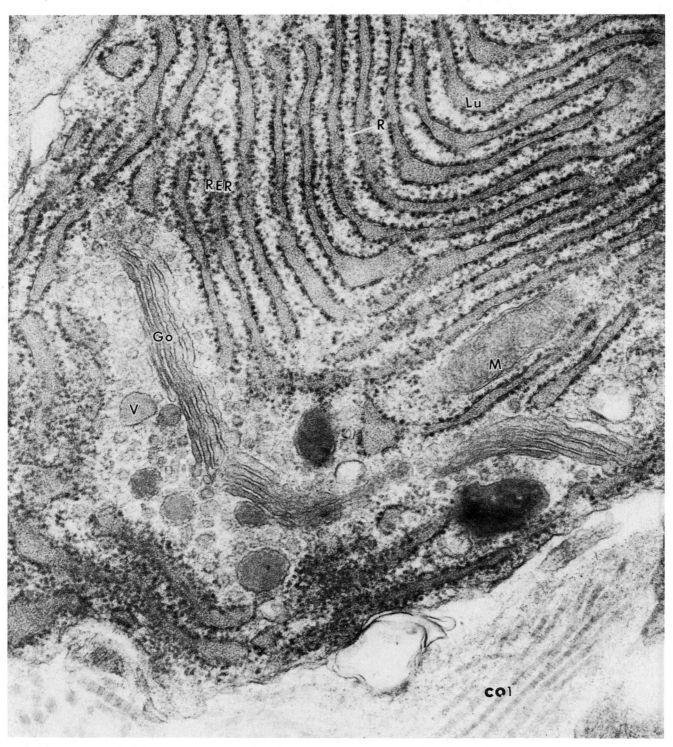

Secretary Organelles

Go—Golgi	rER—Rough Endoplasmic
V—Secretory vesicle	M—Mitochondrla
R—Ribosome	Ci—C
Lu—E.R. Lumen	Pancreatic Acinar Cell

Figure 1.4 Golgi apparatus: Go = Golgi saccule; Psg = pro-secretory granule; sg = secretory granule.

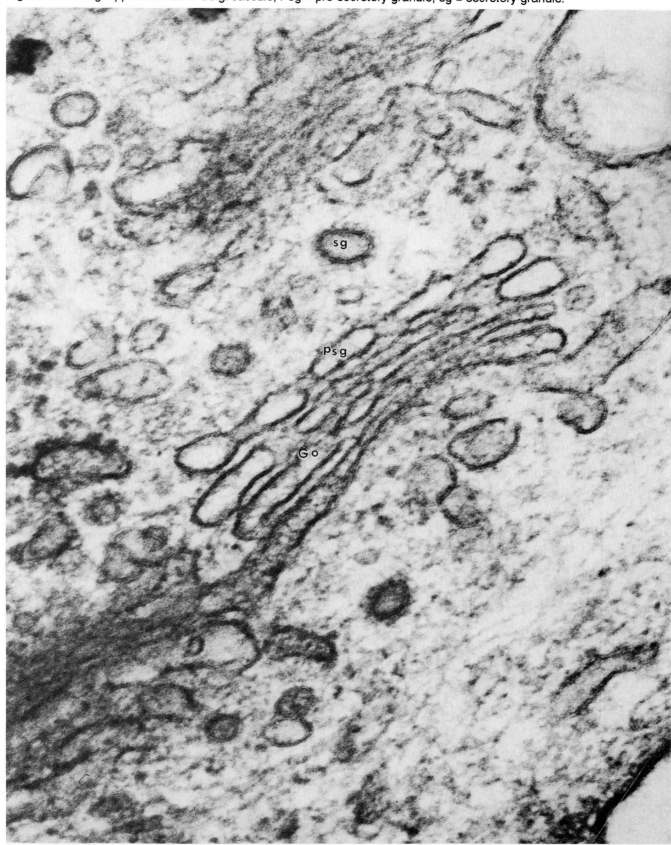

Lysosomes are spherical, membrane-bound organelles 0.2–0.4 nm in diameter. They are involved in intracellular digestion and their appearance is related to their functional state. Lysosomes contain hydrolases such as acid phosphatase, proteases, nucleases, glycosidases, phospholipases, and sulfatases. Lysosomes are present in all cells except erythrocytes and are prevalent in macrophages, osteoclasts, neutrophils, kidney proximal tubule cells, and liver cells. They play an essential role in cellular defense mechanisms and also in the replacement of cellular components and organelles.

Mitochondria appear in light microscopy as spheres, rods, ovoid, or threadlike, cytoplasmic organelles that are typically stained by Janus green B. They were first described by Altmann and Benda in the 1890s. However, their very existence was not completely confirmed until the advent of electron microscopy. Mitochondrial size will range from 0.5 to 1.0 μm in diameter to 5 to 8 μm in length. Their number is related to the energy requirements of the cell with few represented in small lymphocytes but many in hepatocytes and in cells of the stomach, kidney tubules, cardiac muscle, and adrenal cortex. They are usually concentrated in parts of cells that have highest energy requirements and they also appear to move and change shape in an active cell. They are the major source of cellular adenosine triphosphate (ATP).

Electron microscopy reveals that they are generally ovoid structures bounded by a 6 nm-thick outer and inner membrane respectively. The membranes are separated from each other by an intermembranous space 8 nm thick. The outer membrane is permeable to most small ions, whereas the inner membrane, which is arranged into numerous folds, or cristae, is highly selective. The inner membrane can actively transport metabolites into and out of the mitochondrial matrix. The surface areas of the cristae provide a structural surface for oxidative enzymes associated with electron transport and phosphorylation. The mitochondrial matrix contains granules that serve as binding sites for calcium and also contains RNA, circular DNA, ribosomes, and enzymes of the Krebs cycle (fig. 1.1).

Before the very existence of mitochondria was confirmed, some investigators speculated that the mitochondria represented symbiotic bacteria. It is interesting to note that since mitochondria are now known to be semiautonomous organelles containing DNA, RNA, and ribosomes, they resemble bacteria and may have actually originated as aerobic bacteria that became incorporated into evolving animal cells.

Typical Cell

Label illustration using terms listed below.

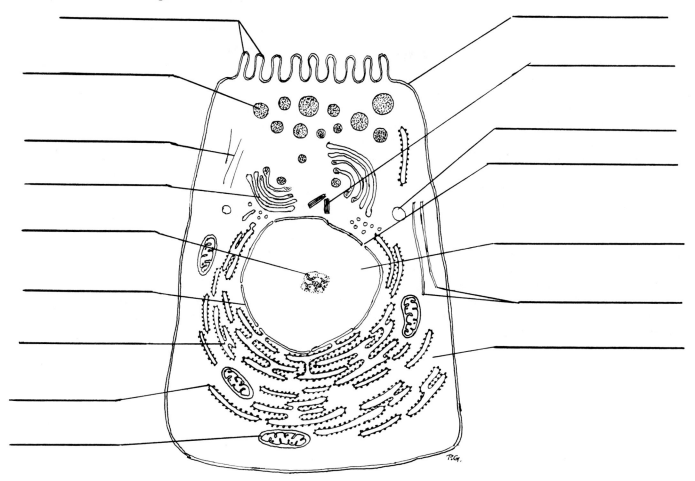

centriole	microtubules	plasma membrane
cytoplasm	microvilli	ribosomes
Golgi complex	mitochondria	secretory granules
granular endoplasmic	nuclear envelope	
reticulum	nuclear pore	
lysosome	nucleolus	
microfilaments	nucleus	

Slides

Examine the following cell types and make drawings in the spaces provided:

1. egg cell, c.s. (mammal)
2. sperm cell (smear)
3. nerve cell, c.s.
4. fat cell, c.s. osmic acid
5. glandular cell (e.g., acinar cell of pancreas)
6. striated muscle cell
7. cell stained for mitochondria
8. cell stained for Golgi bodies
9. blood smears (amphibian and mammalian)

Supply the following labels for each cell type:

1. egg cell: ovum, nucleus, nucleolus, corona radiata, cumulus oophorus, follicular cavity, theca interna, theca externa
2. sperm cell: head, middle piece, tail
3. nerve cell: nucleus, dendrite, axon hillock, Nissl bodies, perikaryon
4. fat cell: nucleus, fat cytoplasmic deposits
5. glandular pancreatic acinar cell: nucleus, basal lamina, zymogen granules
6. striated muscle cell: sarcomere, A-band, I-band, nucleus
7. mitochondria: H&E (oil imm.)
8. Golgi bodies: silver H&E; stomach, small intestine, or spinal cord
9. Blood smear: Wright's stain; RBC, nucleus of RBC, WBC

Draw the following cell types.

Egg cell	Sperm cell
Nerve cell	Fat cell

Glandular cell of pancreas

Striated muscle cell

Mitochondria

Golgi bodies

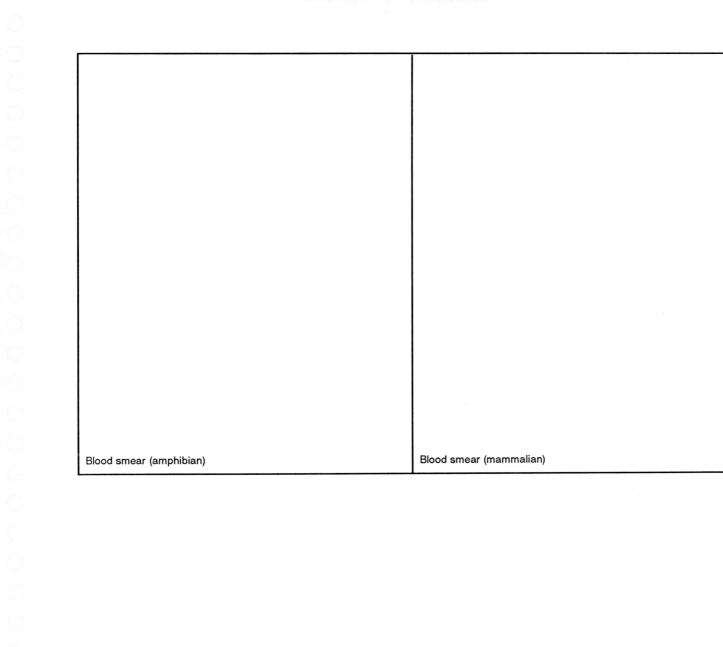

Blood smear (amphibian)

Blood smear (mammalian)

Questions: The Cell

1. Which cells connect the ovum to the follicle?

2. Are the corona radiata cells of the ovum present at fertilization?

3. Is the sperm head similar or different in various mammals?

4. Nissl bodies of neurons are composed of _____.

5. Fat cells are stained by _____.

6. Pancreatic acinar cells secrete _____.

7. What is the average length of a sarcomere in striated muscle?

8. A supravital dye that stains mitochondria is _____.

9. Filamentous mitochondria may be as long as _____ micrometers.

10. Golgi bodies are typically found in what type of cells?

Chapter 2

Epithelial Tissue

Epithelial tissues are arranged in sheets or layers, covering the surface or lining the cavities of the body. They are usually composed of closely aggregated cells lacking protoplasmic processes except for microvilli. Epithelial tissues contain little intercellular substance. Adhesion of the cells is strong, and they are held together by specialized portions of their cell surfaces known as junctional complexes, or cell junctions.

Cell junctions are observed in electron microscopy and are classified according to shape and the proximity of their membranes to adjacent cells. The type known as *tight junctions,* or *zona occludens,* form a girdle of fused membrane of occluding ridges and are usually seen near the terminal or apical border of a cell. These junctions serve to seal and regulate paracellular permeability. They are commonly found in intestinal epithelia. A second type, the *gap junction,* or *nexus,* which is not unique to epithelial tissues, has a narrow intercellular gap between the contiguous cell membranes. The gap is about 2 nm wide and is bridged by small tubular passageways that offer communication between adjacent cells. They facilitate very rapid conduction of transcellular materials and are found in heart muscle and in smooth muscle of the intestine.

A third type is the *adhering junction,* which represents very strong adhesion between contiguous cells. This type is also not restricted to epithelial tissue. In the adhering junction there is no direct contact between unit membranes. The intercellular space is about 20 nm wide.

The adhering junctions are further subdivided into the *belt desmosome,* or *zonula adherens,* and the *spot desmosome,* or *macula adherens.* The belt desmosome forms a band around epithelial cells on the basal side of the tight junction. The spot desmosome is a disc-shaped structure and contains *tonofilaments,* a type of intermediate filament composed of prekeratin, which are anchored to the spot desmosome. *Hemidesmosomes,* or half desmosomes, may occur on the basal surfaces of epithelial cells and serve to join epithelial cells to the underlying basal lamina and connective tissue of the epidermis (fig. 2.1).

Microvilli are narrow cylindrical protoplasmic processes that project from the surfaces of most epithelia. They range in size from about 0.1 μm wide to 2 μm long. In light microscopy, they are identified as the striated border on intestinal epithelia or the brush border of absorptive cells of the proximal convoluted tubule or of the choroid plexus or placental epithelium. The free surface of a cell may contain as many as two thousand microvilli. Each microvillus has a slender core of actin containing fine filaments that anchor at the base and extend into a terminal web. The surface of microvilli contains glycosaminoglycans and as a result they stain periodic acid-Schiff (PAS) positive. Microvilli will increase cell surface area and will function in active transport (fig. 2.2).

Epithelial tissues are derived from all three of the primary embryonic germ layers. The epithelium covering the skin and body openings has an ectodermal origin. The linings of the digestive tract, the respiratory system, and the glands of the digestive tract such as the pancreas and liver are derived from endoderm. Other epithelial tissue such as the lining of the kidney is derived from mesoderm.

Epithelial tissue lacks a vascular supply and has no capillaries. Oxygen and nourishment are received by diffusion from the capillary beds close to the epithelium but located in the connective tissues.

Epithelial tissues are bound to underlying connective tissue by a thin structural complex identified by light microscopists for many years as the *basement membrane.* The basement membrane stains deep black in silver preparations because of reticular fibers; however, it stains red in PAS preparations because of polysaccharides. This structure appears thick in H&E preparations such as in the trachea because of the fixed reticular lamina, however, the basement membrane is very thin beneath transitional epithelium and cannot be observed by light microscopy.

Electron microscopy has demonstrated that the basement membrane is composed of an amorphous basal lamina and a reticular lamina containing reticular and collagenous fibers. The amorphous basal lamina or basement lamina is a product of epithelial cells. This layer is 50 – 100 nm thick and is separated from the basal cell membrane by a lucent (clear) region of 50 nm. The basal lamina appears to be attached to the plasmalemma of the basal epithelium cell and may function as a selective filter regulating the movement of macromolecules. The basal lamina is seen not only in epithelial tissues but also in smooth, skeletal, and cardiac muscle in addition to fat cells.

Figure 2.1 Spot desmosome (macula adherens type) from epithelial tissue: PL = plaque; TN = tonofilaments. (x 120,000).

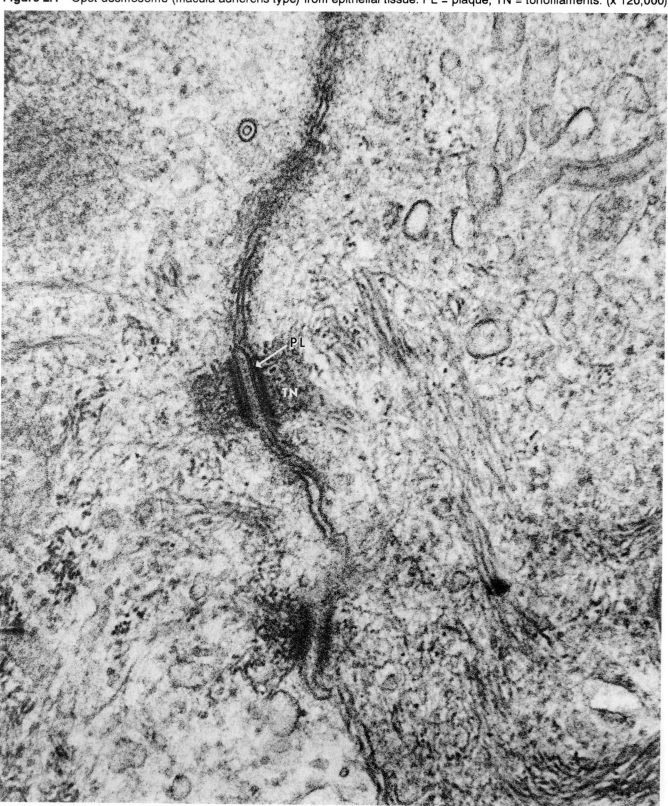

Figure 2.2 Microvilli from proximal tubule of kidney: Mv = microvilli (cross and longitudinal secton) (x 65,000).

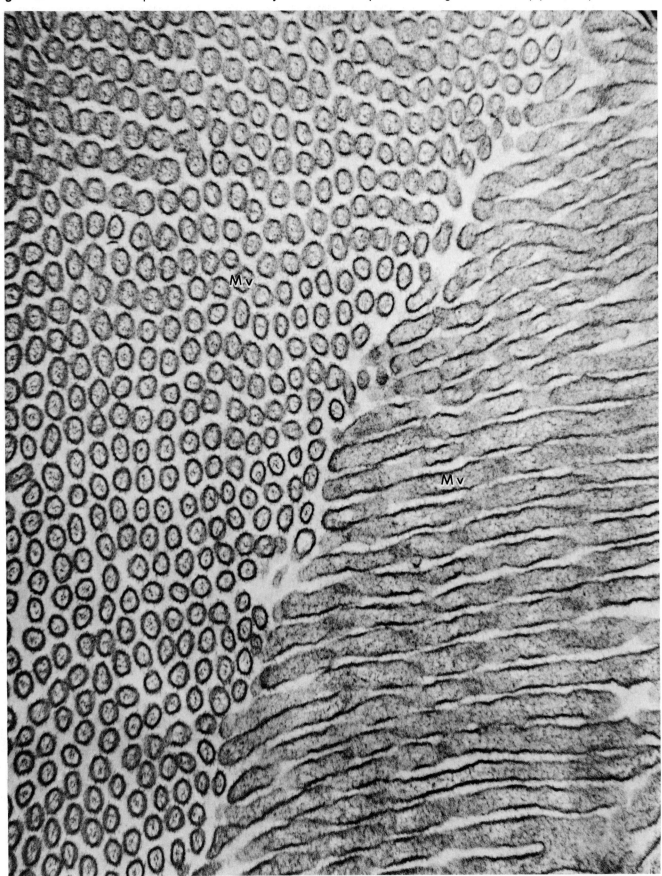

Epithelia can be classed according to the following types: simple epithelia, which consist of a single layer of cells that are in contact with the basement membrane, and stratified epithelia, which consist of cell layers superimposed upon one another and have only the basal layer in contact with the basement membrane. These can be subdivided as follows:

Simple epithelia　*Stratified epithelia*
Squamous　Stratified squamous
Cuboidal　Stratified cuboidal
Columnar　Stratified columnar
Pseudostratified　Transitional

Simple Squamous Epithelium

The cells of *squamous epithelium* are flattened, large, with clear or granular cytoplasm, round, oval, or eccentric nuclei with serrated or smooth cell outlines and with intercellular substance typically stained with silver nitrate. In cross sections the cytoplasm is barely visible. Simple squamous cells are found in barriers where diffusion or filtration, rather than protection, is the basic requirement. Such cells are located in Bowman's capsule of the kidneys and in lung alveoli.

The *endothelium* is a simple squamous epithelium that lines all blood and lymph channels and the heart and bone marrow cavity. Endothelial cells may be phagocytic and can form stellate-shaped connective tissue fibroblasts by cell division.

The *mesothelium* is a serous membrane lining the peritoneal, pleural, and pericardial cavities.

The *mesenchymal epithelium* is a mesothelial-like tissue found lining the anterior chamber of the eye, the inner ear, and cerebrospinal spaces.

The *myoepithelial cells* (basket cells) are cells lying within the basal lamina of glandular acini containing small, dark nuclei and surrounded by a small amount of cytoplasm. Long cytoplasmic extensions reach around the cells of the acinus and are believed to aid in expelling secretion from the gland. They are found in sweat, mammary, salivary, lacrimal, bronchial, and esophageal glands.

In surface view, simple squamous epithelial cells appear as flattened cells with an irregular plasma membrane. This can be demonstrated by the use of silver nitrate stains. The edges of the cells are slightly interdigitated with those of neighboring cells, and the central nuclei are generally spherical or ovoid.

Simple Cuboidal Epithelium

In surface view the cells of *cuboidal epithelium* are smaller and more regular than those of squamous epithelium. In vertical sections the cells appear square-shaped and usually contain a rounded nucleus. These cells may be closely packed around a lumen of some glands and are seen in the lining of kidney tubules and thyroid epithelium.

Simple Columnar Epithelium

Simple columnar epithelium consists of a single layer of cells resting on a basal lamina. In surface view it appears like cuboidal epithelium, however, in sections the cells are taller than broad and are rectangular with the long axis perpendicular to the free surface. This epithelium is the chief secretory and absorptive tissue of the body. The cell nucleus is oval and located close to the base unless the cells are very compressed. The free or apical portion may have a plasma membrane covered with mucus, cilia, or microvilli. A variation of a columnar epithelium cell is the goblet cell. Goblet cells are numerous in the digestive and respiratory tracts and contain mucigen droplets near the apical end. Mucin is formed at the Golgi complex by combining protein components collected at the region of the Golgi complex. Mucigen droplets contain the protein mucopolysaccharide mucin. It is released at the apical end of goblet cells, has adhesive properties, and provides a protective surface for the epithelium.

Pseudostratified Epithelium

The *pseudostratified epithelium* consists of columnar cells crowded very closely together. In cross-section the nuclei appear to be on two or more levels. Because of the crowding, the cells appear distorted and they all do not reach the free surface. However, all of the cells touch the basement membrane. Cells that reach the surface are either ciliated or goblet cells. The goblet cells secrete mucus, which forms a film on the inner surface of the respiratory passages and prevents dust from being inhaled into the lungs. The cilia move the mucus containing the dust particles up and out of the respiratory passages. The cells that do not reach the surface probably serve as progenitor cells producing new cells. Examples of pseudostratified epithelium are found in the upper respiratory tract, the trachea, the male reproductive duct, the Eustachian tube, the pharyngeal portion of the tympanic cavity of the middle ear, and the lacrimal sac of the eye.

Stratified Squamous Epithelium

Stratified squamous epithelium is composed of a basal layer above the basement membrane referred to as the stratum germinativum. Above this layer are several layers of polygonal cells that flatten out and become squamous toward the surface. This epithelium is mainly protective of the organs and tissues that it covers. The number of layers varies considerably in different places. The stratum germinativum contains basophilic, polyhedral cells, which are metabolically active and show considerable mitotic activity. They may contain tonofibrils, which are probably precursors of keratin. Keratin is a tough, resilient material serving a protective function. Examples of moist, nonkeratinized, stratified squamous epithelia are seen in body openings such as the mouth, pharynx, esophagus, auditory canal, and anal, vaginal, and urethral apertures, whereas the skin is composed of keratinized epithelium.

Stratified Cuboidal Epithelium

Stratified cuboidal epithelium contains two or more layers of cuboidal cells. The basement membrane is usually present and the free surfaces have a distinct border. This relatively uncommon type of stratified epithelium is found in the tubules of sweat glands, in the lining of the Graafian follicles, and in the seminiferous tubules.

Stratified Columnar Epithelium

In *stratified columnar epithelium* there is a continuous layer of cuboidal or spherical cells directly on a basement membrane with a columnar layer above. Stratified columnar epithelium is found on wet surfaces where more protection is required than can be afforded by simple columnar epithelium. It is relatively uncommon, but examples may be found in the olfactory mucosa, nasopharynx, larynx, soft palate, and epiglottis.

Transitional Epithelium

Transitional stratified epithelium has a layer of basal columnar cells followed by polygonal cells going toward the surface, which are then followed by pyriform cells and eventually by pear-shaped dome cells, which are convex on their free border. These may appear as squamous cells when the tissue containing this epithelium is stretched. These dome cells may contain numerous mitotic figures, large amounts of DNA, polyploid nuclei and may be binucleated. A basement membrane is not visible in light microscopy and cilia are not found in this type of epithelium. Examples of transitional epithelium are found in the urinary bladder, ureter, a portion of the urethra, renal pelvis, and calyces.

Location of Epithelial Tissues

Simple Squamous

    tympanic membrane
    Bowman's capsule
    pulmonary alveoli
    descending loop of Henle
    posterior cornea
    rete testis
    endothelium of blood vessels, heart and lymph
        vessels, lining of sinusoids of liver
    mesothelium serous membranes lining peritoneal,
        pleural, pericardial cavities
    mesenchymal epithelium lining subarachnoid space,
        anterior eye chambers, and perilymphatic space

Simple Cuboidal

    thyroid
    kidney tubules
    ducts of urinary glands
    choroid plexus
    capsule of lens

Pseudostratified columnar

    parotid gland duct
    male urethra

Pseudostratified Ciliated Columnar

trachea, bronchi
Eustachian tube
tympanic cavity of middle ear
lacrimal sac
male sex ducts

Transitional

urinary bladder
renal calyces
ureter
proximal urethra

Stratified Squamous

skin epidermis (keratinized)
conjunctiva
oral, vaginal, anal, and urethral apertures
external auditory canal
tear ducts, esophagus
pigmented layer of retina
liver parenchyma
germinal surface of ovary

Simple Columnar

lining of digestive tube
excretory ducts of glands
organ of Corti sensory cells
gall bladder
proximal and distal convoluted tubes of kidney

Simple Columnar (Ciliated)

uterus
oviduct
bronchi
some paranasal sinuses
central canal spinal cord
epididymis (stereocilia)
mouth, pharynx

Stratified Cuboidal

excretory ducts, sweat glands
lining of developing ovarian follicles, seminiferous
  tubules

Stratified Columnar

nasopharynx, larynx
epiglottis
ductus deferens
urethra

Stratified Columnar (Ciliated)

nasal surface soft palate
larynx
fetal esophagus

Epithelia

Match the epithelia listed below with the correct illustrations.

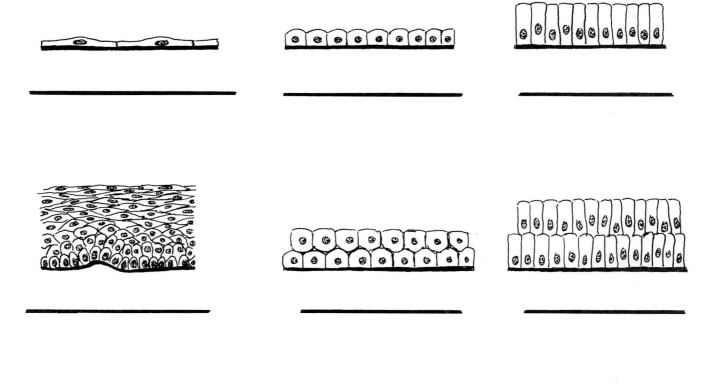

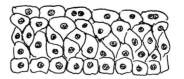

pseudostratified ciliated columnar
simple columnar
simple cuboidal
simple squamous
stratified columnar
stratified cuboidal
stratified squamous
transitional

Slides

Examine the following epithelial tissues and make drawings in the spaces provided:

1. Simple squamous, frog, flat mount, silver or H&E
2. Simple squamous, mammal, Bowman's capsule, c.s., H&E
3. Simple cuboidal kidney, collecting duct or thyroid, c.s.
4. Simple columnar, kidney secreting tubule,ileum, c.s., H&E.
5. Pseudostratified ciliated columnar, trachea, c.s., H&E
6. Goblet cells, intestine, c.s., Masson
7. Stratified columnar ciliated, frog esophagus or mammal epiglottis, c.s.
8. Transitional, rabbit, ureter, c.s., H&E
9. Stratified squamous, dog or rabbit esophagus, skin, c.s., H&E
10. Mesothelium, mesentery, w.m., silver
11. Endothelium, mesenteric vessels, w.m., silver
12. Mesenchyme, frog or pig embryo, c.s., H&E

Supply the following labels for each drawing:

1. Simple squamous: nucleus, cytoplasm, cell membrane, intercellular substance
2. Simple squamous: nucleus, cytoplasm, cell membrane, basement membrane
3. Simple cuboidal: nucleus, cytoplasm cell membrane, basement membrane
4. Simple columnar: nucleus, columnar cell, basement membrane lamina propria
5. Pseudostratified ciliated columnar: nucleus, basal cell, goblet cell, cilia, basement membrane, lamina propria
6. Goblet cells: goblet cell, nucleus, mucigen granules
7. Stratified columnar ciliated : columnar cells, cuboidal cells, basement membrane, cilia
8. Transitional: dome, polygonal, basal and binucleated cells
9. Stratified squamous: squamous, polygonal and basal cells, dividing cells, basement membrane, keratinized skin cells
10. Mesothelium: nucleus, cytoplasm, cell membrane, basement membrane
11. Endothelium: nucleus, cytoplasm, cell membrane, basement membrane
12. Mesenchyme: nucleus, cytoplasm, stellate cell membrane

Draw the following tissues.

Simple squamous (frog)	Simple squamous (mammal)
Simple cuboidal (kidney or thyroid) (C.S.)	Simple columnar (kidney) (C.S.)

Pseudostratified ciliated columnar

Goblet Cells

Stratified columnar ciliated (C.S.)

Transitional (C.S.)

Stratified squamous (C.S.)

Mesothelium (W.M.)

Endothelium (W.M.)

Mesenchyme (C.S.)

Questions: Epithelial Tissue

1. Can cuboidal epithelia change to columnar epithelia and vice versa?

2. Do all cells of pseudostratified endothelium touch the apical surface?

3. Goblet cells form _____ droplets.

4. What type of endothelium can keratinize?

5. The generative layer of endothelium is _____ .

6. The trachea is lined with _____ .

7. Polyploid nuclei may be found in _____ cells.

8. Endothelium, mesothelium, and mesenchyme are all types of endothelium and all are derived from _____ .

9. The basement membrane stains black in silver preparation because of the presence of _____ .

10. The lining of the gall bladder consists of _____ .

Chapter 3

Connective Tissues

Connective tissues, also referred to as mesenchymal tissue, have a common origin from the embryonic germ layer, the *mesoderm. Mesenchyme* is a loose connective tissue component composed of loose stellate and spindle-shaped cells embedded in an intercellular amorphous compound that in this case contains only a few fibers. Mesenchymal cells have multiple developmental potentials and can give rise to any of the connective tissues. Connective tissues differ from epithelial tissues by the presence of abundant intercellular substance.

Cells of connective tissue lie more or less scattered and usually are not in contact with each other, while other times they touch only at the ends of long protoplasmic processes. The intercellular substance is prominent and becomes the most important part of the majority of the tissues. This intercellular substance is also called ground substance or amorphous component and is composed of a colloidal gel of varying viscosity. The cell shape is often stellate with a vesicular nucleus and a cytoplasm that is granular and part of elongated processes. The intercellular components of connective tissue are (1) fibers, (2) ground substance, and (3) tissue fluid. Connective tissue functions to hold other tissues together, that is to bind and/or separate; to give the body support; to transport metabolites; to store energy-rich lipids, water, and electrolytes; to protect against pathogenic organisms, mechanical deformation, and trauma; and to repair damage to its own substance and that of organs it supports or encloses.

Classification of Connective Tissue

A. Connective Tissue Proper: General
  1. Loose Connective Tissue
      a. Mesenchyme: embryonic tissue with stellate cells and amorphous compound
      b. Mucous connective tissue: embryonic mesenchyme tissue in umbilicus (Wharton's jelly)
      c. Areolar: in spaces between muscle fibers and muscle sheaths (fascia); supports epithelial tissue; encircles lymphatic and blood vessels; dermis; serous lining of pleural and peritoneal cavities; and in glands and mucous membranes
      d. Adipose: subcutaneous, omentum, and around organs
      e. Connective tissue fibers
          (1) Collagenous or white fibers: dermis of skin, tendons
          (2) Reticular fibers: lymphatic organs, red bone marrow
          (3) Yellow elastic fibers: ligaments, arteries, cartilage
      f. Connective tissue cells: most types seen in areolar tissue
          (1) Fibroblasts
          (2) Histiocytes or macrophages
          (3) Mast cells
          (4) Fat cells
          (5) Plasma cells
  2. Dense Connective Tissue
      a. Collagenous: tendons (attaching muscle to bone), dermis
      b. Elastic: yellow ligaments of vertebral column
B. Supporting Connective Tissue: Specialized Connective Tissues
  1. Precartilage
      a. Chondroid: precartilage of embryo
      b. Notochord: replaced by vertebral column
  2. Cartilage
      a. Hyaline: trachea, nose, larynx, bronchi
      b. Elastic: external ear, Eustachian tube, epiglottis, larynx
      c. Fibrous: intervertebral discs, ligaments and tendon attachments, pubic symphysis

            d. Articular: hyaline-type at articular surface of bone
    3. Bone
            a. Cancellous (spongy): flat bones of skull, epiphysis
            b. Compact: diaphysis of long bones
    4. Joints
            a. Synarthrosis (poorly moveable)
                    (1) Syndesmosis: skull
                    (2) Synchondrosis: epiphyseal discs
                    (3) Synostoses: fused syndesmosis and synchondrosis
            b. Diarthrosis (freely moveable)
                    (1) Symphyses: pubic symphysis
                    (2) Synovial: articulating bones
    C. Hemopoietic Connective Tissue
    1. Lymphatic: lymph nodes, thymus, spleen, tonsils and Peyer's patches
    2. Myeloid tissue: bone marrow
    3. Blood: leucocytes and erythrocytes

Fibers of Connective Tissue

Collagenous or White Fibers

Collagenous fibers are very common and found in the corium or the dermis and in most areolar tissue. These fibers are arranged in bundles of indefinite length and thicknesses varying from 10 to 100 μm or more. The bundles are composed of fibers 1–12 μm in diameter. These fibers are in turn composed of fibrils observable by light microscopy with diameters from 0.2 to 0.5 μm. These fibrils are composed of smaller fibrils described in electron microscopy, ranging from 20 to 200 nm. These in turn are composed of microfibrils 3–15 nm in diameter.

The microfibrils are composed of tropocollagen molecules, 1.5 nm wide and 280 nm in length. These macromolecules are composed of three polypeptide chains in the form of a coiled helix. The polypeptide chains can differ individually in their amino acid sequences rendering the collagen macromolecules different in various parts of the body. The electron microscope shows fibrils of mature collagen to exhibit an axial periodicity with cross bandings at intervals of 64 nm. Collagenous and reticular fibers arise extracellularly by polymerization of procollagen to collagen molecules secreted into the ground substance by fibroblasts (fig. 3.1).

Reticular Fibers

Reticular fibers are similar to collagenous fibers that form a network, exhibit a similar axial periodicity of 64 nm, do not stain with eosin but with silver salts, and are argyrophilic. In addition, they stain more darkly with the periodic acid-Schiff (PAS) staining technique compared to collagenous fibers, which is apparently due to the presence of carbohydrate on the surface of each fibril. Some investigators believe that reticular fibers are immature collagen fibers since they have the same 64 nm cross banding and are morphologically and biochemically similar except for diameter. They are found as fine networks around small blood vessels, adipose cells, and muscle and nerve fibers and at boundaries between connective tissue and other types of tissue such as liver tissue. Reticular fibers also form dense networks as components of basal laminae beneath epithelial tissues.

Yellow Elastic Fibers

Yellow elastic fibers have a smaller diameter than collagenous fibers and reach a diameter of 10 – 12 μm. They may occur singly or may be arranged as branches, bundles, or sheets. Elastic fibers contain the amorphous albuminoid protein elastin, which is released upon boiling. However, elastic fibers are extremely resistent to weak acids, alkalis, and moderate heat. These fibers do not show axial periodicity. However, the elastin acquires a fibrous shape because of microfibrils within and on the periphery of the fiber. Yellow elastic fibers are found in arteries and ligaments and may occur singly, branching, in bundles, or in sheets. These fibers show no cross banding and are readily stained by resorcin. They are also found in areolar connective tissue and have their origin in fibroblasts. Elastic fibers show a decrease in elasticity in aging due to surface changes associated with the glycosaminoglycans (GAGS), the principle component of ground substance.

Figure 3.1 Collagen: Col = collagen fibril (x 160,000).

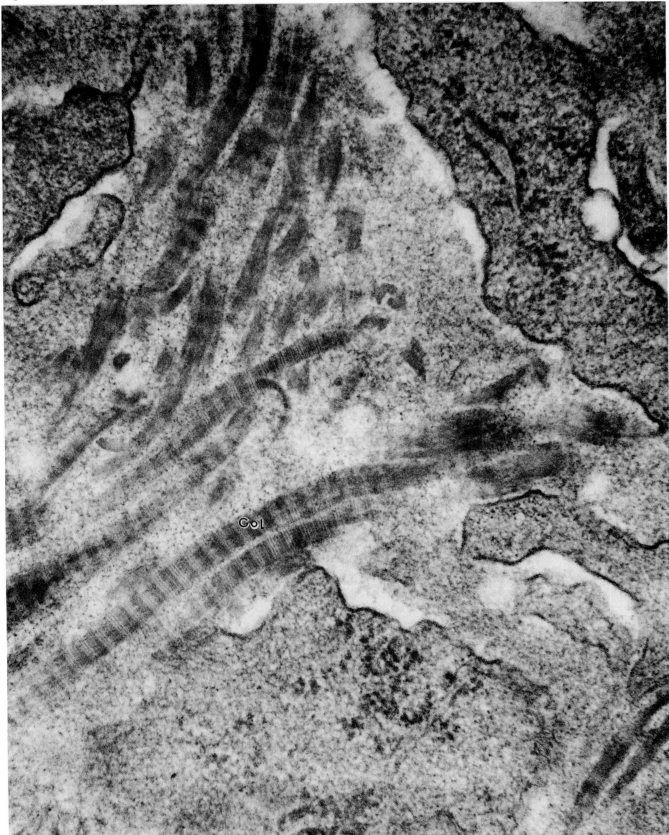

Collagen

Ground Substance

Ground substance is a noncellular, nonfibrous material forming the matrix of connective tissue. It is composed of acid mucopolysaccharides, more accurately referred to as glycosaminoglycans (GAGS), which contain hyaluronic acid, chondroitin sulfate, keratin sulfate, and in mast cells, heparin. Electron microscopy has demonstrated that intercellular fibers of ground substance are elaborated by modified portions of the endoplasmic reticulum and the Golgi complex.

Lamina Propria

Beneath the mucosa layer of the digestive tube is a layer of loose areolar connective tissue consisting of a delicate network of collagenous and reticular fibers, a few fibroblasts and plasma cells. This is the *lamina propria*. Scattered lymphocytes, plasma cells, mast cells, and white blood cells are also present. Isolated lymphatic nodules are common, and in the ileum these nodules are numerous and aggregate into large masses of lymphoid tissue often visible to the naked eye. These aggregated nodules are termed *Peyer's patches*. There is evidence that Peyer's patches may be homologous to the bursa of Fabricius, a hind gut diverticulum in birds, since they are involved in the development of lymphoid cells (B-lymphocytes), which are capable of transformation into (immunoglobulin) antibody-producing plasma cells.

Basal Lamina

For many years light microscopy has revealed an extracellular layer under the basal surface of epithelial cells that was identified as the basement membrane. Its presence was demonstrated by staining with the PAS reaction or with silver impregnation methods. Electron microscopy has revealed that what was formerly identified as the basement membrane is not a membrane and consists of two or more components, the *basal lamina* (or basement lamina) and the *reticular lamina* (lamina reticularis). The basal lamina is in contact with the basal plasma membrane of the epithelial cells and is a sheet of extracellular fibrillar material (50–80 nm thick) containing ground substance and polysaccharides that are stained by PAS reagents. On the connective tissue side there are fine reticular fibers and microfibrils of collagen. This layer is identified as the reticular lamina, which is readily stained with silver salts. Basal laminae act as diffusion barriers to rapid ion exchanges and also provide a strong connection between epithelia and underlying connective tissue.

Cells of Loose Connective Tissue

Fibroblasts

Fibroblasts are the most common connective tissue cells, have their origin in mesenchyme, and occur in all types of fibrillar tissue such as areolar tissue. These cells are considered responsible for the formation of connective tissue fibers and are thought to elaborate most, if not all, of the intercellular substance. Fibroblasts have abundant basophilic cytoplasm, well-developed granular endoplasmic reticulum and Golgi complex; weakly stained ovoid nucleus with chromatin granules; numerous mitochondria near the nucleus; and an elongated and stellate shape. The branching processes are long and slender. Young fibroblasts, which are actively engaged in protein synthesis for the production of intercellular substance, demonstrate a homogenous and basophilic cytoplasm because of the abundant granular endoplasmic reticulum. Older and relatively inactive fibroblasts have little endoplasmic reticulum and weakly basophilic cytoplasm and are called *fibrocytes*. In the formation of collagen, amino acids such as glycine and proline are collected on the ribosomes of the granular endoplasmic reticulum and transported to the Golgi complex. Subsequently, procollagen is formed that polymerizes extracellularly to form the collagen fibril.

Macrophages (histiocytes)

Macrophages are oval or spherical cells in fibrous tissue that are capable of rapid movement and phagocytosis. They have small nuclei that are darkly stained and indented on one side as compared to nuclei of fibroblasts. They contain cytoplasm with numerous vacuoles and granules. They originate from monocytes that enter loose connective tissue. Macrophages are active in the inflammatory process and are part of the macrophage (reticuloendothelial) system. These cells act as scavengers to help rid the body of harmful invaders. Recently, macrophages have also been shown to play a crucial role in the healing of wounds. They are often found in cancer tissue and in some cases appear to attack cancer cells. In addition, they are often present near atherosclerotic plaques that are a crucial factor in heart disease. In addition, viruses that cause AIDS and bacteria that cause leprosy and legionnaire's disease can survive in macrophages. Macrophages exert their healing, growth promoting, and sometimes killing effects by means of recently identified substances such as transforming growth factors, platelet derived growth factor, and insulinlike growth factor. These substances are believed to help attract more macrophages to clean a wound of debris, kill invading bacteria, replace cells, repair tissue, and promote development of blood vessels to restore blood supply.

Mast Cells

Mast cells were identified by Ehrlich in 1879 and are large, round cells with somewhat small central and pale nuclei. The cytoplasm has many basophilic granules. These granules contain primarily histamine and the anticoagulant heparin. Mast cells resemble basophilic leucocytes of the blood. Mast cell granules are membrane bound and can be displayed with use of basic dyes such as toluidine blue. In addition, electron microscopy reveals well-developed Golgi apparatus but few mitochondria and ribosomes. The histamine released by the mast cell granules may promote anaphylaxis by causing capillaries to dilate and to leak plasma thus causing edema of the surrounding tissues. This reaction may be initiated when antibodies attach to mast cells and, in the presence of allergens, stimulate the release of histamine by the mast cells. Mast cells develop from mesenchyme cells and are numerous in the connective tissues of the skin and mucous membranes. They are also distributed chiefly in the vicinity of small blood vessels, thymus, and to a lesser degree in other lymphatic organs.

Fat Cells (adipocytes)

Fat cells store fat and form no intercellular fibers or matrix. They are mesenchymal in origin and develop as fat deposited in the cytoplasm as droplets that coalesce to occupy most of the substance of the cell. The nucleus is compressed and flattened along the edge of the fat cell giving the cell a signet ring appearance. In H&E sections, fat cells appear as empty cavities whereas in osmic acid preparations, the fat resists the action of alcohols and will appear as a deeply stained mass occupying the center of each cell. In the preparation it is stained black. Sudan dyes will also stain the fat in fat cells a black color. There is no intercellular substance elaborated by adipose tissue cells. They normally lie embedded in reticular or areolar tissue.

Plasma Cells

Plasma cells are comparatively rare in most connective tissue but are fairly common in the tunica propria as lymphatic nodules of the digestive tract, in the greater omentum, and in reticular connective tissues of blood-forming organs. Their number is greatly increased in areas of chronic inflammation. This is related to the fact that plasma cells are the major producers of circulating antibodies, which are synthesized within the granular endoplasmic reticulum. They are formed from hematopoietic stem cells and from B-lymphocytes. The cells are ovoid, about 10 μm in diameter with small eccentric nuclei. The chromatin material in the nucleus is concentrically arranged like a cartwheel. The cytoplasm is basophilic and rich in granular endoplasmic reticulum with a large Golgi complex and centrioles.

Areolar Connective Tissue

Label illustration using terms below.

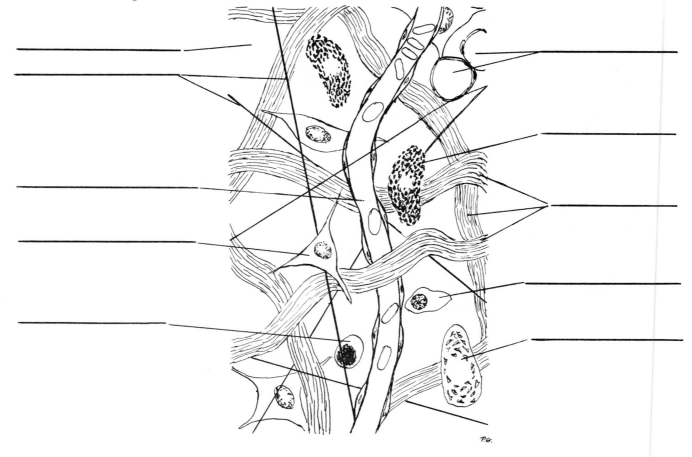

adipose cell
capillary
collagenous fibers
elastic fibers
ground substance
macrophage
lymphocyte
mast cell
plasma cell

Slides

Examine the following loose connective tissues:

1. Collagenous tissue, h.p. and oil.
2. Reticular tissue, silver, h.p.
3. Yellow elastic tissue, h.p.
4. Areolar tissue (general) with fibers, h.p. (collagenous fibers)
5. Areolar tissue cells—oil
    a. Fibroblast
    b. Mast cell
    c. Macrophage
    d. Plasma cell
    e. Fat cell

Supply the following labels for each drawing:

1. Collagenous tissue: bundles, fibers, fibrils (oil)
2. Reticular tissue: netlike fibers (black)
3. Yellow elastic tissue: fibers (red)
4. Areolar tissues: collagenous fibers, elastic fibers, fibroblasts, histiocytes, fat cells
5. Areolar tissue cells–oil
    a. Fibroblast: pale nucleus, stellate-shaped cells, cytoplasm
    b. Mast cell: nucleus, basophilic granules
    c. Macrophage: nucleus, vacuoles, granules
    d. Plasma cell: nucleus (eccentric, cartwheel), Golgi, centrioles
    e. Fat cell: nucleus, fat droplet

Draw the following tissues.

Collagenous tissue (h.p.)	Collagenous tissue (oil)
Reticular tissue (h.p.)	Yellow elastic tissue (h.p.)

Areolar tissue (h.p.)

Areolar tissue (oil)

Fibroblast (areolar tissue—oil)

Mast cell (areolar tissue—oil)

Macrophages (areolar tissue—oil)

Plasma cell (areolar tissue—oil)

Fat cell (areolar tissue—oil)

Questions: Connective Tissues

1. Collagen is a _____ and stains with most dyes.

2. Collagen fibers yield _____ on boiling and are a source of _____ (commercial material).

3. Vitamin _____ is necessary for collagen formation.

4. Cartilage changes associated with aging involve a decrease in the (chemical component) _____ and an increase in _____ proteins.

5. Mucopolysaccharides are sulfated and _____. The type are generally more _____.

6. Reticular fibers can best be stained with _____ or _____.

7. Reticular fibers are composed mainly of the protein _____.

8. Elastic fibers are composed of the scleroprotein _____ and are stained by _____.

9. Mucopolysaccharides of the intercellular matrix are secreted primarily by _____ cells.

10. Fibroblasts develop from _____ cells, where active ones demonstrate a _____ cytoplasm, while relatively inactive ones demonstrate _____ cytoplasm.

11. In an area of inflammation, histiocytes are seen engulfing _____ cells that died in the process of engulfing and destroying bacteria.

12. Macrophages can easily be identified in sections of tissue from animals injected with _____ or _____.

13. Mast cell granules contain the sulfated mucopolysaccharide _____.

14. Antibodies attached to mast cells will stimulate the mast cell granules to liberate _____ and _____.

15. Mast cells stain metachromatically with toluidine blue because _____.

16. Plasma cells originate from _____ cells and when stimulated will secrete _____.

17. Plasma cell cytoplasm is _____ and the nuclear chromatin has a _____ appearance.

Chapter 4

Supporting Connective Tissue: Cartilage, Bone, and Joints

Cartilage is a connective tissue that contains cells, fibers, and ground substance. The ground substance in cartilage is composed primarily of chondromucoids containing abundant chondroitin sulfate; in bone, the ground substance is impregnated with inorganic salts such as calcium phosphate. The fetal skeleton of vertebrates is composed of cartilage. Although most of the embryonic cartilage is replaced by bone by a process called *endochondral ossification,* cartilage persists in the articular surfaces of bones, larynx, trachea, ear, nose, and intervertebral discs.

The histogenesis of connective tissue involves the stellate mesenchymal cells retracting their protoplasmic extensions, becoming round, and multiplying rapidly forming condensed agglomerations. These cells are now chondroblasts with basophilic cytoplasm. Subsequently, matrix formation separates the groups of cells while surrounded by a condensed matrix.

Growth may be *interstitial,* which is early growth due to mitotic division of preexisting chondrocytes, or *appositional* in mature cartilage where cartilage increase is due to the addition of new layers at the periphery by the perichondrium.

Cartilage contains no blood vessels, nerves, or lymphatic vessels, and nourishment is by diffusion from capillaries into adjacent connective tissue or by synovial fluid from joint cavities.

Cartilage

Three types of cartilage are hyaline, elastic, and fibro cartilage.

Hyaline cartilage is the most common and has a clear or glasslike appearance. It contains dispersed collagenous fibers throughout the tissue in a fine network filled in by ground substance containing collagen and proteoglycans, a macromolecule composed of GAGS linked to a protein. In ordinary staining the fibers and matrix are indistinguishable. However, after digestion of the ground substance or by silver impregnation or polarized light or under electron microscopy, the fibers become distinguishable. Age changes possibly caused by poor nutrition result in a thickening of cartilages with the homogenous matrix replaced by closely packed coarse fibers. Such changes are due to a decrease of acid mucopolysaccharides and an increase in noncollagenous proteins. Calcification of the matrix is also seen in old cartilage and associated degenerative changes of cartilage cells.

The cartilage cells (*chondrocytes*) lie centrally within mature hyaline cartilage, are large, and tend to be arranged in groups or cell nests. The chondrocytes occupy matrix spaces called lacunae. The matrix appears homogenous and stains blue-gray with H&E. Chondrocytes near the perichondrium are smaller and individually arranged. The *perichondrium* is composed of an outer fibrous layer, which contains fibroblasts that produce the collagen resulting in the characteristic fibers, and an inner chondrogenic layer containing chondroblasts that deposit new cartilage matrix.

Examples of hyaline cartilage are found in the nose, larynx, trachea, bronchi, fetal skeleton, and articular surface of most joints.

Elastic cartilage is similar to hyaline cartilage in that in addition to collagenous fibers it contains an abundant network of fine elastic fibers. Elastic cartilage has a yellowish color when fresh, which is caused by the presence of elastin in the elastic fibers. The elastic fibers may be seen by special staining such as Verhoeff's elastic stain. The chondrocytes are large within the interior and tend to be smaller toward the perichondrium. Elastic cartilage is more opaque and flexible than hyaline cartilage and is not prone to degeneration or calcification. Examples of elastic cartilage are in the epiglottis, Eustachian tubes, external auditory canal, and some of the laryngeal cartilages.

Fibrocartilage has structural characteristics intermediate between those of dense connective tissue and hyaline cartilage. The chondrocytes are present either singly or in small groups and are very often arranged in long columns. There is little ground substance and the matrix is acidophilic because it contains a great number of highly interwoven collagenous fibers that impart great strength and that stain red with eosin. A perichondrium is generally lacking in the adult. Examples of fibrocartilage are found in attachments of certain ligaments to bones, in the pubic symphysis, and in the intervertebral discs.

Bone

Unlike epithelial tissue and other connective tissue, *bone* forms a complete system of supporting tissues, namely the skeleton. It consists of cells and matrix with the matrix composed of densely packed collagen fibrils infiltrated with calcium mineral salts. There is little ground substance. The *osteocytes* (bone cells) have adopted a different form than chondrocytes. They have developed long processes extending through fine passages throughout the matrix called *canaliculi*. The cell bodies lie in a large cavity, the *lacuna*. The cells and fibers are organized in concentric circles called *lamellae*.

Bone is one of the hardest tissues of the human body and is composed of an intercellular calcified material, the bone matrix, and osteocytes that are found within lacunae (cavities) embedded in the matrix. In addition there are bone-building cells called *osteoblasts* and bone resorbing cells called *osteoclasts*. Osteoblasts are rounded or pyramidal-shaped cells with an eccentric nucleus, deeply basophilic cytoplasm, and much rER. Osteoblasts are frequently arranged in a continuous layer in an epithelial-like arrangement and are typically found between the periosteum and developed bone.

Osteoclasts are involved in the resorption of bone. Mineral is deposited in the matrix in the form of calcium hydroxyapatite crystals. These crystals lie alongside the collagenous fibers and are surrounded by amorphous ground substance. Compact bone has a lamellar arrangement. The lamellae of bone matrix, the cells, and the central canal constitute the Haversian system, or osteon, the unit of structure of compact bone.

There are four types of lamellar arrangements.

1. *External circumferential lamellae* extend around the periphery of bone laid down by the osteogenic cells of the periosteum.
2. *Internal circumferential lamellae* are found in the interior regions of bone and resemble external circumferential lamellae in arrangement and appearance. They are laid down by the endosteum which lines the marrow, or medullary cavity.
3. *Concentric lamellae* are internal to the above and constitute small channels around which the bony substance is laid down in concentric plates. They run parallel to the long axis of the bone. The central canal is known as the *Haversian canal* and contains blood vessels, lymph vessels, and nerves. They are joined laterally and obliquely to one another by *Volkmann's canals*.
4. *Interstitial lamellae* are nonconcentric lamellae and they lie between the Haversian system (concentric lamellae and Haversian canals) and remnants of old Haversian systems. If concentric lamellae were removed leaving only interstitial lamellae, we would have spongy bone. Passing from the interstitial and circumferential lamellae to the periosteum are coarse collagenous bundles known as *Sharpey's fibers*. These fibers serve to firmly anchor the periosteum to the bone especially at regions of insertion of ligaments and tendons.

Bone is surrounded by *periosteum,* which is a connective tissue made up of collagenous and elastic fibers and is found on all bone surfaces except articular surfaces. The periosteum has two layers: (1) the outer fibrous layer which is a thin, dense connective tissue layer with fibroblasts and blood vessels; and (2) the inner osteogenic layer, which contains flat, spindle-shaped osteoblasts in addition to the periosteal collagenous fibers, Sharpey's fibers.

In embryonic development, bone follows one of two methods of bone formation (ossification): *intramembranous* (direct) or *endochondral* (intracartilaginous or indirect). In intramembranous bone formation, as in the flat bones of the skull, a mesenchymal sheet or membrane becomes vascular with cells developing into osteoblasts. A matrix develops, which subsequently calcifies, and is deposited around the osteoblasts. In endochondral bone formation, as seen in the long bones, the cartilage model grows by interstitial and appositional growth and becomes vascularized, and cells of the perichondrium become osteoblasts. Osteoblast activity is stimulated by the thyroid hormone *thyrocalcitonin.*

Bone is vascular and grows by having new bone developed on its surface by appositional growth. However, as new bone is added to this exterior surface, bone must be resorbed from its inner surface so that the lumen may increase in diameter. The resorption of bone is performed by osteoclasts. Osteoclasts are located in small concavities on the surface of bone known as Howship's lacunae. Osteoclasts are multinucleated and may contain up to 12 nuclei with a basophilic cytoplasm containing many vacuoles and lysosomes. These cells are responsive to parathormone of the parathyroid glands, which stimulates the release of lysosomal enzymes involved in bone resorption.

Joints

The bones are joined together to form the skeleton by a series of articulations, the structure of each varying with the degree of moveability of the joint. It has been stated that diseases of the joints constitute the greatest single cause of disability encountered by the medical profession. Joints may (1) permit articulation between two bones, (2) become as solid as the bones they connect, and (3) make it possible for structures that connect to grow in extent.

Joints may be classified according to embryonic development, type of movement (physiological), or type of structure (morphological).

Structural and Functional Classification

Synarthrosis (Poorly Moveable Joints)

Syndesmoses is a type of articulation that permits a certain limited amount of movement and bones are joined by fibers of elastic connective tissue such as the inferior tibiofibular articulation or the sutures of the cranial bones of a young skull. Subsequent bone growth may replace connective tissue sutures with bone transforming the syndesmosis to a synostosis.

Synchondrosis is a type of articulation in which bones are joined by hyaline cartilage that is nearest the bone and subsequently by fibrous cartilage. Examples are seen in the epiphyseal discs since they contain hyaline cartilage connecting portions of bones; in intervertebral discs, which contain fibrocartilage surrounding the notochord remnant, nucleus pulposus; and the attachments of ribs to the sternum.

Synostosis is a type of articulation in which bones are united by bony tissue and no movement takes place. Examples are seen in the skull bones of the adult.

Diarthrosis (Freely Moveable Joints)

Symphysis is a type or articulation that may also be classified as a synchondrosis since the ends of bone are capped with hyaline cartilage and followed by fibrous tissue blending with the hyaline cartilage. An example of this is the pubic symphysis, which consists largely of fibrocartilage and which is controlled by the hormones relaxin and estrogen. In late pregnancy there is marked pelvic relaxation as the pubic symphysis increases in vascularity followed by imbibition of water, disaggregation of fibers and depolymerization of the mucoproteins in the ground substance. These changes are due to the action of the hormone relaxin in conjunction with estrogen.

Synovial joints are articulations that are freely moveable and located between long bones. They contain a joint capsule, a colorless, transparent, viscous fluid rich in hyaluronic acid called the synovial fluid. The joint capsule contains two layers, an outer, fibrous layer and an inner layer making up the synovial membrane. The inner lining of the synovial membrane contains squamous and cuboidal cells, which lie over dense connective tissue, plus adipose tissue and blood vessels. The cells covering the synovial membrane synthesize hyaluronic acid and proteins, which make up the synovial fluid.

Types of Cartilage

Label illustrations using terms listed below.

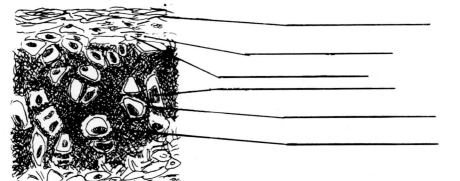

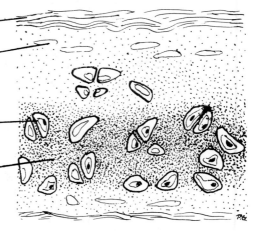

3 Types of Cartilage

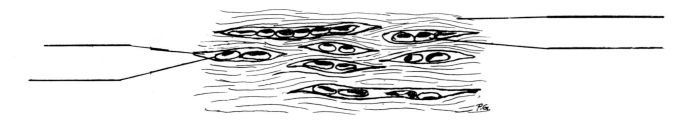

Elastic cartilage

chondroblast
chondrocyte
elastic fibers (matrix)
lacuna
perichondrium

Fibrocartilage

chondrocyte
collagenous fibers
lacuna
matrix

Hyaline cartilage

chondroblast
chondrocyte
lacuna
matrix
perichondrium

Bone

Label illustration using terms listed below.

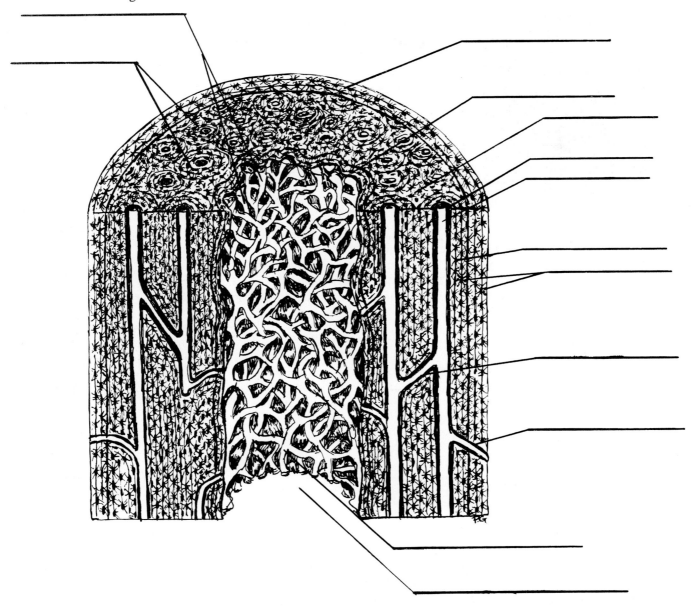

Bone (c.s. and l.s.)

interstitial lamellae
marrow cavity
perforating canal
periosteal (external lamellae)
spongy bone
trabeculae
Volkmann's canal

canaliculi
capillary
concentric lamellae
endosteal (internal) lamellae
Haversian canal
lacuna

Slides

Examine the following supporting connective tissues and make drawings in spaces provided:

1. Notochord tissue, c.s.
2. Chondroid tissue (decalcified phalange of human embryo)
3. Hyaline cartilage, l.p., c.s., H&E
4. Elastic cartilage, l.p., c.s., Verhoeff's stain
5. Fibrocartilage, l.p., H&E
6. Bone, decalcified, compact, H&E
7. Bone, ground, c.s.
8. Bone, ground, l.s.

Supply the following labels for each drawing:

1. Notochord tissue: vacuolated cells, peripheral cells
2. Chondroid tissue: mesenchyme
3. Hyaline cartilage: chondrocyte, nucleus, vacuole, lacuna, perichondrium (inner chondrogenic layer–outer fibrous layer), matrix
4. Elastic cartilage: chondrocyte, lacuna, perichondrium, elastic fibers, matrix
5. Fibrocartilage: chondrocyte, lacuna, perichondrium fibers
6. Bone, decalcified: lacunae, osteocytes, yellow marrow, periosteum
7. Bone, ground, c.s.: Haversian system, canal, lamellae, periosteum, and osteone
8. Bone, ground, l.s.: Haversian system, canal, lamellae, periosteum, Volkmann's canal

Draw the following tissue.

Notochord tissue	Chondroid tissue
Hyaline cartilage	Elastic cartilage

Fibrocartilage

Bone, decalcified

Bone, ground (c.s.)

Bone, ground (l.s.)

Questions: Supporting Connective Tissue

1. Metabolic and nutritive materials are exchanged in cartilage by _____ .

2. In fixed preparations chondrocytes are greatly vacuolated and shrunken into small masses separated by spaces from the walls of the lacunae. Why? _____ .

3. Cartilage growth may be _____ or _____ .

4. Perichondrium consists of two layers, the _____ and _____ .

5. Hyaline cartilage is typically found in _____ and _____ .

6. Chondrocytes of fibrocartilage are usually arranged _____ .

7. Haversian canals contain _____, _____, and _____ .

8. In ossification, periosteal buds containing _____, _____, and _____ invade _____ .

9. The articular surface of bones in synovial joints is lines with _____ _____ .

10. The synovial fluid contains a water binding mucopolysaccharide called _____, which is secreted by the _____ cells covering the synovial membrane.

Chapter 5

Blood and Blood Formation

Mesenchyme, the embryonic connective tissue, will in addition to giving rise to connective tissue proper, cartilage, and bone, also give rise to blood, lymph, and blood vessels. The fluid portion of blood or the lymph comprises the intercellular substance whereas the blood cells represent free connective tissue since blood cells are not attached to other cells or held in position by intercellular substances.

Red Blood Corpuscles (RBC) or Erythrocytes

Erythrocytes perform their function within the blood, whereas white blood corpuscles (WBC), or leucocytes, generally perform their function when they leave the blood and enter loose connective tissue or other tissues. Under normal conditions the erythrocyte count of males is 5.2 million per cubic millimeter and 4.5 million per cubic millimeter in females. A normal leucocyte count is 5,000 – 9,000 per cubic millimeter in a healthy adult. Fresh preparations of RBC appear greenish or straw-colored. However, they are typically stained by Wright stain and range from 7 to 7.5 μm in size.

Mature RBCs in adult mammals lack nucleus, endoplasmic reticulum (ER), Golgi, and centrioles; are biconcave discs; and range in size from 9 to 12 μm as macrocytes but some called microcytes may be smaller than 6μ m. In hypotonic solutions they undergo *hemolysis* by absorbing water and swelling, and they assume a spherical shape with hemoglobin passing through the cell membrane resulting in an empty-looking cell often referred to as a "ghost cell." In hypertonic solutions they undergo *crenation* by losing water and shrinking. The average life span of an RBC is about 120 days, after which it is removed by macrophages by phagocytosis (figs. 5.1 and 5.2).

White Blood Corpuscles (Leucocytes)

The colorless *leucocytes,* or *white blood corpuscles,* are "true" cells and contain a nucleus and cell organelles. They exhibit a limited amount of amoeboid movement and are divided according to their granularity.

Granular Leucocytes

Granular Leucocytes comprise 60–70% of WBC and contain a multilobed nucleus.

Neutrophils (Polymorphs)

Neutrophils comprise 60 – 70% of leucocytes and are 10 – 12 μm in diameter. The nucleus has two to five lobes that are separated by fine strands. The nucleus is highly polymorphous and has basophilic chromatin, which stains blue or purple with Wright's stain. A *Barr body* (condensed x chromosome), or "drum stick," appears as a chromatin appendage in one out of 38 (or about 3%) of neutrophils in females. The cytoplasm contains very fine neutrophilic granules, which give the cytoplasm a lavender (lilac) color with Wright's stain. These neutrophilic granules are a special type of lysosome containing hydrolytic enzymes that are liberated during phagocytosis. Neutrophils are motile and pass through blood vessels into tissues to phagocytize bacteria, especially during inflammation.

Eosinophils (Acidophilic Leucocytes)

Eosinophils comprise 1 to 4% of WBC and range between 10 to 15 μm in diameter. The nucleus is bilobed with a cytoplasm containing coarse granules that stain pink to bright red. Eosinophils are weakly phagocytic, are motile, and can enter tissue. They increase in number as a result of an allergic reaction in the body such as occurs during parasitic infections. They are believed to function in selective phagocytosis of antigen-antibody complexes. They also may function in blood clot prevention by secreting profibrinolysin. Since hydrocortisone depresses allergic reactions, eosinophils will disappear from the blood after cortisol treatment.

Figure 5.1 Scanning electron micrograph (S.E.M.) of oopen capillary showing erythrocytes: Ery = erythrocyte; Col = collagen.

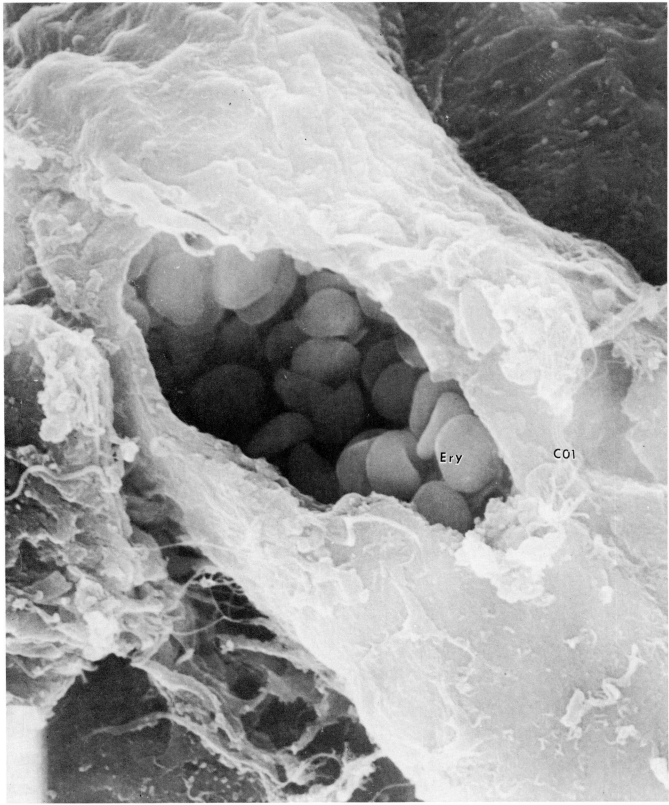

Blood Vessel   Ec—erythrocyte
CS.E.M.   Ci—Collagen

Figure 5.2 Erythrocytes: P = plasma; Ery = erythrocyte; Eb = erythroblast; Pt = platelet; En = endothelium; BM = basement membrane.

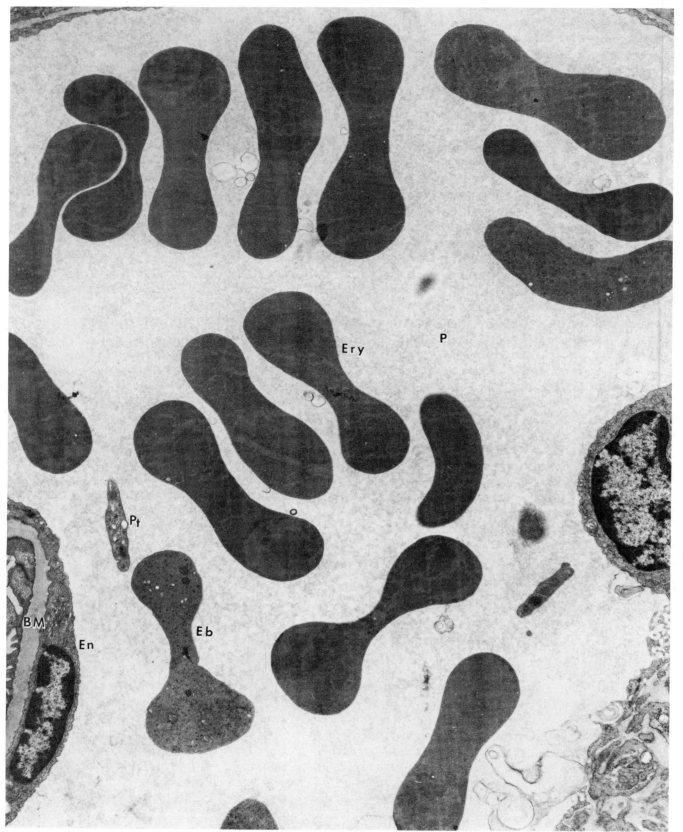

Basophils

Basophils comprise 0.5–1.0% of WBC and range from 10 to 12 μm in diameter. The nucleus is often S-shaped with a constriction in two or more regions. The cytoplasm contains large, dark-blue stained granules that are similar to those of mast cells. The granules contain histamine and anticlotting mucopolysaccharides such as heparin. Mitochondria and Golgi are also present. Basophils are capable of amoeboid movement and phagocytosis, they may leave the blood stream as a result of hormonal (cortisone) action, and they are apparently involved in allergic and inflammatory phenomena. Their role in allergic reactions is controversial.

Nongranular Leucocytes

Lymphocytes

Lymphocytes comprise 20–30% of leucocytes. These cells fall into two size categories, a small type ranging from 5 to 8 μm and a large type ranging from 10 to 12 μm. The nucleus is large, round or oval, and indented on one side. Nucleoli are seen in well-prepared thin sections. The cytoplasm is homogenous, basophilic with many ribosomes and with occasional purple azurophilic granules at the periphery with few mitochondria and with Golgi at the outer side of the centriole.

The small lymphocytes are separated into two types, B-lymphocytes and T-lymphocytes.

B-lymphocytes: B-lymphocytes are short-lived lymphocytes that originate from bone marrow stem cells. They migrate into the general circulation in mammals and subsequently into gut-associated lymphoid tissue (GALT) such as Peyer's patches in the ileum, tonsils, and the vermiform appendix. They are called B-lymphocytes because they were first identified in the bursa of Fabricius (a hind gut diverticulum in birds). They are short-lived in that their life span is up to several months in man.

B-lymphocytes are associated with humoral immunity. Electron microscopy reveals a large number of filamentous projections on the surface that are antibody receptors and are associated with the production of antibodies such as immunoglobulins. When a foreign antigen reacts with the receptors on the B-lymphocyte surface, an immunoglobulin molecule surface complex is formed, which enters the cell by pinocytosis. This triggers the conversion of a B-lymphocyte to a plasma cell that will in turn secrete antibodies. These antibodies will attach to mast cells, which when stimulated will liberate histamine and heparin in the intercellular spaces.

T-lymphocytes: T-lymphocytes constitute 80% of the circulating lymphocytes in humans and are long-lived in that they survive for months or years. These lymphocytes are associated with cell-mediated immune reactions including foreign graft rejection. They originate from bone marrow stem cells, and via the circulation reach the thymus therefore giving rise to their name. They move from the capsule of the thymus to the cortex and then differentiate into T-cells. Upon leaving the thymus, via the circulation, they may also reenter peripheral lymphoid organs or they may also return to the bone marrow. T-cells are programmed to react with particular antigens and form into several subsets such as natural "killer" cells, suppressor, and/or helper T-cells.

Monocytes

Monocytes comprise 3–8% of leucocytes. They resemble lymphocytes and are the largest leucocytes with sizes ranging from 12 to 15 μm in diameter. The nucleus is usually large, oval, and slightly indented, horseshoe-shaped, twisted, and folded, with a fine chromatin that stains a pale blue-violet color with Wright's stain. Two nucleoli are seen in phase contrast microscopy. The cytoplasm is well represented and stains a blue-gray color. Azurophilic granules, which are probably lysosomes containing enzymes, are observed in the cytoplasm in addition to mitochondria and Golgi apparatus.

Monocytes are motile and migrate through capillaries or small venules entering loose connective tissue to become phagocytotic macrophages. It is believed that they may also give rise to fibroblasts. Monocytes originate from hematopoietic stem cells in the bone marrow, and they have a life span of about three days.

Platelets

Blood platelets arise from giant cells in the bone marrow called *megakaryocytes.* Blood platelets are rounded or ovoid, colorless, protoplasmic discs 2–5 μm in diameter. They number 200,000 to 300,000 per cubic millimeter of blood. In profile they appear spindle or rod-shaped. They are lacking in lower vertebrates where they are essentially represented by thrombocytes.

Leucocytes

Label illustrations using terms listed below.

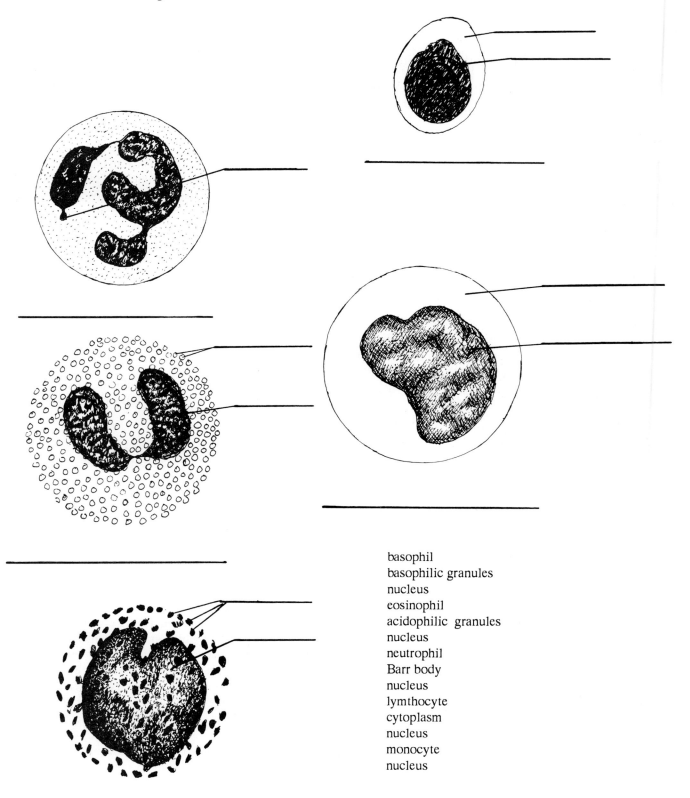

basophil
basophilic granules
nucleus
eosinophil
acidophilic granules
nucleus
neutrophil
Barr body
nucleus
lymthocyte
cytoplasm
nucleus
monocyte
nucleus

Platelets demonstrate two regions: a centrally located basophilic granular zone, the granulomere, containing vesicles, mitochondria, and dense granules; and a pale, homogenous peripheral zone, the hyalomere, devoid of organelles except microfilaments. Platelets arise from megakaryocytes and presumably produce the enzyme *thromboplastin,* which aids in the transformation of prothrombin into thrombin in the clotting reaction. Thrombin in turn transforms fibrinogen into fibrin. The vasoconstrictor serotonin is also found in platelets.

Megakaryocytes are giant cells in the bone marrow derived from hemocytoblasts. These cells will range from 30 to 100 μm in diameter and give rise to blood platelets. The nucleus is lobulated with many connecting thin strands and is polyploid containing 32n to 64n chromosomes. The cytoplasm contains fine granules and Golgi apparatus. It has been demonstrated that platelets arise from fragmentation of pseudopodia of the megakaryocytes.

Slides

Examine the following blood slides and make drawings in spaces provided:

1. Frog blood smear, Geimsa
2. Camel blood smear, Geimsa
3. Human blood smear, H&E
    a. Neutrophil
    b. Eosinophil
    c. Basophil
    d. Lymphocyte
    e. Monocyte

Supply the following labels for each drawing:

1. Frog blood: nucleated erythrocytes, leucocytes
2. Camel blood: elliptical erythrocytes, leucocytes
3. Human neutrophil: chromatin, neutrophilic granules, Barr body (if present)
4. Human eosinophil: chromatin, eosinophilic granules
5. Human basophil: chromatin, basophilic granules
6. Human lymphocyte: indented nucleus, nucleoli, clear cytoplasm
7. Human monocyte: indented nucleus, fine chromatin, blue-gray cytoplasm

Draw the following from blood slides.

Blood (frog)	Blood (camel)
Neutrophil (human blood)	Eosinophil (human blood)

Basophil (human blood)

Lymphocyte (human blood)

Monocyte (human blood)

Hemopoietic Organs

The development of red blood cells in the adult is normally limited to the bone marrow. However, in the embryo, red blood cells will develop from extra embryonic mesoderm of the yolk sac and subsequently from the liver and spleen. In addition, granular leukocytes are developed from stem cells in the embryonic bone marrow referred to as *myeloblasts,* or *hematocytoblast* cells. The origin of lymphocytes is bone marrow stem cells and their development is mediated by the thymus in case of the T-cells and through GALT (gut-associated lymphoid tissue) in the case of B-cells.

Blood formation mediated by the bone marrow and not by lymphatic tissues is referred to as *myelopoieses.* Bone marrow consists primarily of red marrow, which contains a framework of reticular tissue or stroma with fat cells, blood cells, and capillaries. Sinusoids are present as wide, tubular channels lined with endothelial cells (littoral cells). Bone marrow will contain the following cell types:

Hematocytoblast (myeloblasts, stem cell). These cells are 10 – 12 μm diameter, have a basophilic nongranular cytoplasm, are pear-shaped or polygonal with no protoplasmic processes, and have a large nucleus. The following are derivatives of the hematocytoblast.

The cells of the *erythrocyte series* are:

a. *Proerythroblast cells,* which are 10 – 15 μm in diameter; have a fine, granular chromatin with two nucleoli and a weakly basophilic cytoplasm
b. *Basophilic erythroblast cells,* which are smaller cells with more condensed chromatin and basophilic cytoplasm
c. *Polychromatic erythroblasts,* which have basophilic cytoplasm and polyribosomes indicating hemoglobin synthesis. The cytoplasm stains greenish gray-violet with Giemsa stain and there is a smaller nucleus course chromatin.
d. *Normoblasts* have loose, cytoplasmic basophilia and a small, pyknotic nucleus that is later extruded and phagocytosed giving rise to an enucleated red blood cell.

The *granulocyte series* consists of:

a. *Myeloblasts,* which are 15 – 20 μm in diameter with a large, spherical nucleus with fine chromatin and one or two nucleoli. The cytoplasm is slightly basophilic.
b. *Promyelocytes,* which are large cells ranging up to 20 μm in diameter with a rounded or ovoid nucleus that is occasionally indented. The cytoplasm is granular and nucleoli are prominent. The cytoplasm is basophilic and contains azurophilic granules. Electron micrographs show numerous mitochondria, a well-developed Golgi, and reticulum.
c. *Myelocytes* develop from the promyelocytes and are subdivided into three types:
   1. *neutrophilic myelocytes,* which give rise to the neutrophilic leukocytes
   2. *eosinophilic myelocytes,* which give rise to the eosinophilic leukocytes
   3. *basophilic myelocytes,* that give rise to the basophilic leukocytes

Hemopoiesis

Label illustration using terms listed below.

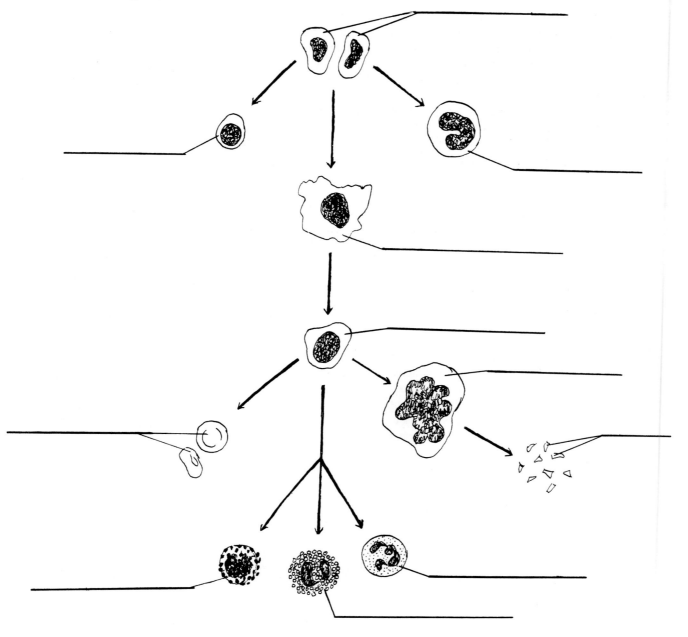

basophil
eosinophil
erythrocytes
hematocyte stem cells
lymphocyte
megakaryocyte

monocyte
neutrophil
platelets
primitive
reticular cell

Slides

Examine the following:

1. Bone marrow, H&E

   Supply the following drawings and necessary labels in spaces provided:

1. Myeloblast: large nucleus, nucleoli, basophilic cytoplasm
2. Basophilic erythroblast: basophilic cytoplasm
3. Polychromatic erythroblast: acidophilic cytoplasm
4. Normoblast: nucleus, cytoplasm
5. Neutrophilic myelocyte: lobed nucleus, neutrophilic granular cytoplasm
6. Eosinophilic myelocyte: lobed nucleus, eosinophilic granules
7. Basophilic myelocyte: nucleus, basophilic granules
8. Megakaryocyte: lobed nucleus, cytoplasmic granules

Draw the following:

Myeloblast (bone marrow)	Basophilic erythroblast
Polychromatic erythoblast	Normoblast

Neutrophilic myelocyte

Eosinophilic myelocyte

Basophilic myelocyte

Megakaryocyte

Questions: Blood and Blood Formation

1. Mature erythrocytes lack a nucleus, Golgi, centrioles, and _____.

2. The most important chemical component of the mature erythrocyte is _____.

3. The average life span of an erythrocyte is about _____ after it is are removed by the _____.

4. In a hypertonic environment, erythrocytes will undergo _____, whereas in a hypotonic environment they will undergo _____.

5. The frequency of the appearance of the Barr body in the neutrophils of females is about _____.

6. The cytoplasm of neutrophils has fine granules that typically stain _____.

7. The nucleus of a neutrophil will usually have _____ to _____ lobes.

8. The eosinophil count will typically increase during _____ infection.

9. The cytoplasmic granules of eosinophils will stain intensely with _____ dyes.

10. The granules of basophils are _____ in size and have an affinity for _____ dyes.

11. B-lymphocytes are formed in _____ and are associated with _____ immunity.

12. T-lymphocytes differentiate in the _____ and are associated with _____ immunity.

13. Electron microscopy reveals filamentous projections on the surface of _____, which are associated with _____.

14. The so-called killer cells associated with graft rejection are actually modified _____.

15. Monocytes range about _____ in size and may enter loose connective tissue to become phagocytic _____.

16. Blood platelets arise from _____.

17. Megakaryocytes are derived from _____ and contain a _____ nucleus.

18. Myeloblasts have a _____ cytoplasm, whereas eosinophilic myelocytes have an _____ cytoplasm.

Chapter 6   Muscle

Early anatomists described muscle after gross dissection as composed of elongated structures they called fibers. With the development of the light microscope and cell theory it became evident that fibers were composed of contractile cells. Contractility is a fundamental characteristic of most tissues. Muscle and nerve are often viewed as the body's two "excitable tissues." In muscle tissue, the properties of contractility and to a lesser degree conductivity have been developed to a great extent. Muscle cells are elongated with many well-defined nuclei. The cytoplasm (sarcoplasm) stains red with eosin and contains fibrils (myofibrils). The cells are surrounded by a limiting plasma membrane (sarcolemma). Muscle fibers are bound in fibroconnective tissue that contains a rich network of blood capillaries to supply oxygen and food materials and also to eliminate waste products. Muscle may terminate in tendons that are anchored in bone or cartilage or they may be attached to periosteum, aponeuroses, or the reticular layer of dermis of the skin.

There are three types of muscle: (1) skeletal/striated/voluntary (controlled directly by the central nervous system), (2) smooth/unstriated/involuntary (controlled by autonomic nervous system), and (3) cardiac/heart/striated (controlled by autonomic nervous system).

Skeletal Muscle

Skeletal muscle originates from embryonic mesoderm giving rise to myoblasts that fuse and give rise to muscle fibers (cells). The central nucleus migrates toward the sarcolemma and becomes eccentric. The fibers (cells) are fusiform and range from 1 to 40 μm long or longer and 10 to 40 μm wide. Many nuclei may be present. The interior of the fiber contains myofibrils that range from 1 to 2 μm in diameter. The cross striations of skeletal muscle are a property of the myofibrils and the striations represent regions of varying refraction. The dark staining band is doubly refractive (birefringent), or *anisotropic,* when studied under polarized light and is referred to as the *A-band.* The light staining band is relatively monorefringent, or *isotropic,* when viewed under polarized light and is known as the *I-band.*

The I-band is bisected by an intermediate disc referred to as the *Z line* (*zwischenscheibe,* from German meaning end line). The A-band is bisected in the *M line,* or middle disc (*mittelscheibe,* from German meaning middle line). On either side of the M line is a pale zone referred to as Hensen's zone. The distance between two Z lines is the *sarcomere,* which is the contractile unit. The myofibrils, which are the smallest contractile elements visible under light microscopy, are shown by electron microscope to be divided into smaller units, the *myofilaments* (fig. 6.1). The myofilaments are in turn divided into two types:

1. thicker filaments containing the protein myosin. These filaments are 11 nm in diameter and 1.5 μm long and make up most of the A-band.
2. thinner filaments containing the protein actin. The thinner filaments are 5–6 nm in diameter and 1 μm in length and extend from the Z line in either direction making up the I-band by extending into part of the A-band.

Muscle fibers may vary in appearance and function and are classified as white (fast or phasic type), red (slow or tonic type), and intermediate. *White fibers* are large, have many myofibrils, much endoplasmic reticulum, little myoglobin, and few mitochondria. Muscles with white fibers contract more rapidly but fatigue quickly. *Red fibers* are smaller, contain numerous mitochondria, are slow acting, and can maintain contractions for longer periods of time. *Intermediate fibers* have structure and function intermediate between the two previously mentioned types. The elongated nuclei of skeletal muscle fibers are located at the periphery of the fibers within the sarcoplasm and just under the sarcolemma. The peripheral location of skeletal muscle nuclei is an outstanding histological characteristic of this tissue as compared to the central location of smooth and cardiac muscle nuclei.

Contraction is due to the action of the thin filaments containing actin moving into the interstices between the thick myosin filaments within which they interdigitate. The thin filaments in addition to containing actin also contain the fibrous protein tropomyosin and a complex protein called troponin. At contraction, calcium ions become available from sacs of the sarcoplasmic reticulum within the myofibril. The calcium ions unite with troponin thus releasing tropomyosin, which

Figure 6.1. Skeletal muscle: SR = sarcoplasmic reticulum; M = mitochondria; A = A-band; I = I-band; H = H-band; Z = Z-line; M = M-line.

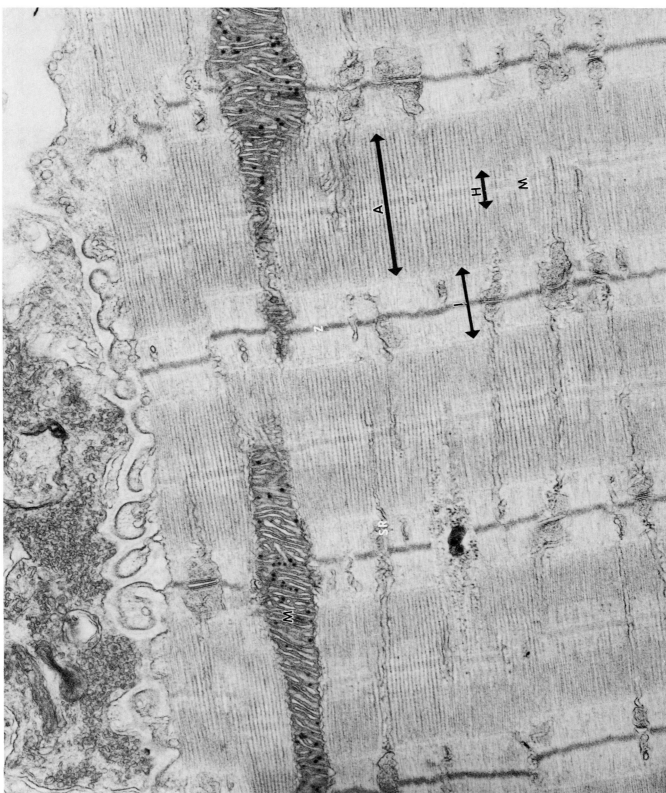

removes the inhibition of the actin-myosin interaction causing the myosin heads of the thick filaments to combine with the actin molecules.

Skeletal muscles are attached to bones through tendons. At regions where muscles join with the tendons there are many nuclei indicating regions of rapid growth. The muscle fibers composing a muscle are gathered in bundles or *fascicles*. A fine, connective tissue called the *endomysium* surrounds the individual fibers. Covering a bundle or fascicle is a connective tissue called *perimysium*. The sheath surrounding a group of bundles is the *epimysium*.

Smooth Muscle

Smooth muscle originates from mesenchyme cells that elongate to a spindle-shaped form containing little intercellular substance. These spindle-shaped cells develop elongated nuclei and are recognized as *myoblasts*. These differentiating muscle cells acquire filamentous contractile elements and their external surface is surrounded by an external lamina that segregates them from the surrounding connective tissue. As in skeletal muscle the term *fiber* is used to denote a single cell.

Mature smooth muscle fibers are spindle-shaped or fusiform and range from 0.02 to 0.5 μm wide by 4 to 7 μm long. The nucleus is central, elongated, and located at the thickest part of the cell. There is no cross banding and the cells are firmly attached by intercellular bridges and tight junctions. At some places they are separated by a basement membrane. The fibers are packed and form a sheet or bundle. Electron microscopy shows that the plasma membrane contains subsurface vesicles that may be pinocytotic. There are perinuclear mitochondria and Golgi with poorly developed, smooth ER.

Smooth muscles are generally located in the viscera as the inner circular and outer longitudinal muscles lining the digestive tract including ducts and glands associated with the digestive system; in arteries, veins, and larger lymphatic vessels; in the dermis of the skin; and in the respiratory, urinary, and genital systems. On the basis of innervation and function, smooth muscle is divided into the *visceral* (unitary) type and *multiunit* type. The visceral type contains relatively few nerve terminals and the stimulus spreads from cell to cell by nexuses (gap junctions). This slower contraction is found in the viscera and small blood vessels. The multiunit type has a rich nerve supply with most, if not all, cells receiving a nerve terminal. In this type the contraction of the cells is very rapid and simultaneous. The multiunit type is seen in the iris of the eye, larger arteries, and the ductus deferens. Smooth muscles are innervated by the sympathetic and parasympathetic branches of the autonomic nervous system.

Cardiac Muscle

Cardiac muscle is involuntary and striated. It is found in the myocardium of the heart. Cardiac muscle has the ability to contract spontaneously without any nerve supply. Contraction is initiated by depolarization of special pacemaker fibers, the *Purkinje fibers,* at the sinoatrial region of the heart. The Purkinje fibers contain mitochondria, glycogen, and few myofibrils but they have more sarcoplasm, are larger in diameter than typical cardiac fibers, and are occasionally binucleate. At the sinoatrial region innervation by the autonomic nervous system regulates the rate of contraction but the heartbeat originates in the pacemaker fibers themselves.

Evidence from light microscopy has suggested that cardiac muscle fibers appear to branch and anastomose extensively to form a syncytial network. However, electron microscopy has demonstrated that the fibers are composed of individual cells joined end to end. The fibers are narrow, ranging from 9 to 11 μm in diameter and are joined end to end by specialized junctional zones 0.05–1 μm thick called *intercalated discs.* The intercalated discs are located at the Z lines and appear in a steplike formation. They contain in the transverse regions spot desmosome-type (macula adherens) cells junctions and in the longitudinal regions gap junctions. These are areas of low electrical resistance permitting rapid impulse conduction between cells resulting in the myocardium serving as a functional but not an anatomical syncytium.

The branching fibers are enclosed in a sarcolemma. One or two centrally located nuclei per cell may be observed. Mitochondria with many cristae are much more abundant than in skeletal muscle and are clustered around the nucleus. Golgi is also located near the nuclear region.

Electron microscope studies show membrane-bound granules, 100–450 nm in diameter in the atria, which are referred to as *atrial granules.* They are more numerous in the walls of the right atrium than the left. The atrial granules are the source of a peptide hormone called atrial natriuretic factor (ANF). Atrial distension results in the release of ANF from the atrial granules resulting in increased renal sodium, potassium, and water excretion. It appears that ANF release is related to regulation of blood pressure and blood volume in addition to aldosterone secretion by the adrenal glands and control centers in the brain that regulate water excretion and blood pressure.

Draw the following from muscle slides.

Smooth muscle (teased)	Smooth muscle (section)
Striated muscle	Striated muscle (c.s.)

Striated muscle (l.s.)

Cardiac muscle (l.s.)

Motor nerve ending

Questions: Muscle

1. The cytoplasm of muscle cells may be referred to as _____ and the plasma membrane as the _____.

2. The location of the nucleus in skeletal muscle fibers is _____ whereas in smooth muscle fibers the nucleus is located _____.

3. The distance between two Z lines comprises a _____.

4. The thick filaments of skeletal muscle contain _____, whereas the thin filaments contain _____.

5. In muscle contraction _____ ions unite with _____ to release _____.

6. In a subsequent stage of muscle contraction, the _____ heads of the _____ filaments will combine with the _____ molecule.

7. A connective tissue sheath surrounding bundles or fascicles of muscle fiber is the _____.

8. In cardiac muscle, adjacent cells are separated by a dark, transverse band known as _____.

9. Cardiac muscle fibers contain a _____ located nucleus and are enclosed in a _____.

10. Atrial granules are the source of _____.

Chapter 7   Nervous Tissue

The nervous system provides for the control and coordination of many of the body's activities. It spreads out widely to all organs from the central nervous system, permitting a multitude of finely graded responses. The nervous system is composed of nerve cells, which have the properties of irritability and conductivity. The nerve cells, or *neurons,* are highly differentiated and hyperirritable, but have lost the power and ability to move and to reproduce. The interstitial tissue of the nervous system is composed of the *neuroglia,* or *glia.* The neuroglia provide support and protection for the neurons and are also thought to assist neurons in their activities in that certain glial cells invest axons with a myelin sheath increasing the speed of impulse conduction. The nervous system is divided anatomically into the *central nervous system* (CNS) comprising the brain and spinal cord and the *peripheral nervous system* (PNS) comprising ganglia, cranial and spinal nerves, and nerve endings including organs of special sense.

Neurons have a cell body called the *perikaryon,* which is the cytoplasmic thickening including the nucleus, or *karyon.* Long processes extending from the perikaryon are the dendrites, which are afferent processes that transmit impulses toward the perikaryon, and the *axon* which is the efferent process that transmits impulses away from the cell body. Neurons may be unipolar when they contain a single fiber that is the axon and no dendrites as seen in sensory ganglia; bipolar when there is one axon and one dendrite as in the retina of the eye; and multipolar, the most common type, when there are several dendrites and only one axon.

The nucleus, or karyon, is large and central, vesicular, lightly stained with a single prominent nucleolus and fine chromatin granules. The cytoplasm is basophilic and contains *Nissl bodies,* or tigroid bodies, which can be stained with toluidine blue or cresyl violet. Electron microscopy has demonstrated that Nissl bodies are clusters of endoplasmic reticulum (ER) and ribosomes and are probably involved in intracellular transport of proteins.

Between the Nissl bodies and in both the axon and dendrites are *microtubules* and *neurofilaments.* The microtubules are 20–30 nm in diameter and are typically interspersed with neurofilaments which are 7 nm in diameter. The neurofilaments are aggregated into neurofibrils which are visible after silver nitrate impregnation. Numerous Golgi are located around the nucleus and mitochondria are abundant in the perikaryon as well as in the dendrites and axons.

Lipofuscin granules begin to appear at an early age and increase in number and distribution with advancing age. They are apparently secondary lysosomes representing the end product of long lysosomal activity and their accumulation is believed to eventually inhibit the normal functioning of some neurons. This represents a normal part of the aging process.

Nerves or nerve trunks of the peripheral nervous system are arranged in groups or bundles of fibers containing axons, dendrites, and their collaterals bound together by connective tissue and invested with blood capillaries. A single bundle of nerve fibers and connective tissue is called a *fascicle.* The *epineurium,* a connective tissue sheath enclosing several fascicles of a nerve trunk, is composed of fibroblasts, collagenous and elastic fibers. The *perineurium* is composed of collagenous fibers concentrically arranged and surrounding a single fascicle. It may be thick in large nerves and thin in smaller nerves. The *endoneurium* is composed of branches of the perineurium, which penetrate the fascicle and in turn separate the individual nerve fibers.

Nerve fibers are divided into four histological types: (1) fibers without observable sheaths (e.g., gray matter of the spinal cord), (2) fibers with prominent fatty myelin sheaths (e.g., white matter), (3) fibers with a sheath enclosing only a minute quantity of myelin (e.g., nonmyelinated fibers of the autonomic nervous system), and (4) fibers with a cellular sheath enclosing a thick layer of myelin (e.g., white fibers of PNS).

The *axon,* typically the neuron's longest nerve fiber, is single and usually arises from an enlarged portion of the neuron termed the *axon hillock.* The body of the axon is composed of the axis cylinder containing argyrophilic neurofibrils embedded in neuroplasm or axoplasm. The diameter of the axon can range from less than 1 μm to 20 μm, while the length may range from less than 1 mm to 1 m or more. The axon will end in twiglike branchings, the telodendria, which reach the next cell body, dendrites, or axons of one or more neurons at a specialized neurotransmitter containing and ending termed the *synapse.*

The *myelin sheath* is a phospholipid containing component that stains black with osmic acid and is also stained by PAS test indicating a carbohydrate component. The myelin sheath is actually the spirally disposed plasma membrane of the Schwann cell folded and laminated to provide a highly resistant sleeve of insulation around the axon. The myelin sheath is interrupted at regular intervals leaving the axolemma bare. The gaps are referred to as the nodes of Ranvier. The segment between two nodes is the internode. The myelin of each internode is covered by a Schwann cell that lies end to end along a myelinated and an unmyelinated fiber. A myelin sheath is found in myelinated fibers of the PNS and in the white matter of the brain and spinal cord (fig. 7.1).

Afferent Sensory Nerve Fibers

Afferent nerve fibers are divided into somatic afferent and visceral afferent.

Sensory endings of afferent neurons are subdivided into (1) specialized endings of the eye and ear, (2) free nonencapsulated endings, (3) encapsulated endings, and (4) muscle spindles. Specialized nerve endings are bare nerve endings as seen in the cornea of the eye. Free and nonencapsulated endings, which are the most common and are terminal branches of delicate fibers, often show a slight enlargement. They are found in practically all parts of the body in connective tissue, muscle, and other serous membranes. Encapsulated endings contain a central naked fiber or several branches embedded in tissue fluid and enclosed within a connective tissue capsule. Types of encapsulated endings are as follows.

1. Tactile corpuscles of Meissner lie within the connective tissue of a dermal papilla and are oval structures composed of flattened connective tissue cells in the form of horizontal lamellae surrounded by a connective tissue capsule. Two or more myelinated nerve fibers reach the corpuscle where the myelin sheath disappears with a naked axon passing into the corpuscle and with a branch and spiral within the connective tissue. These tactile corpuscles are found on the lips, fingers, eyelids, and external genitalia.
2. Bulbous and cylindrical corpuscles are the corpuscles of Krause, which are spheroidal in shape and contain modified Schwann cells and nerve endings along a transverse axis. They are located in the mucocutaneous areas in the dermis of the lips and external genitalia. These endings are sensitive to cold. The spindle-shaped corpuscles of Ruffini are sensitive to heat, contain a central core of collagen, and terminal branches of nerve fibers. They are located in connective tissue and joint capsules, and are found deep in the dermis especially on the plantar surface of the feet.
3. The lamellar and oval-shaped corpuscles of Pacini (Vater-Pacini) are relatively large structures 2 mm in length, 0.5 to 1 mm in diameter containing a large number of concentric lamellae with each lamella consisting of connective tissue fibers lined by a single layer of flat connective tissue cells. The lamellae are separated from one another by a clear fluid. Each Pacinian corpuscle is supplied by a single myelinated nerve fiber. A naked axon extends through the center of the inner bulb terminating in a knoblike expansion.
4. Muscle spindle sensory nerves terminate in slender bundles of muscle fibers as complicated end organs called muscle spindles. The terminal parts of the nerve fibers are arranged spirally around the muscle cells. Connective tissues and blood vessels are included with the muscle and nerve fibers and all are enclosed in a connective tissue capsule. Within the capsule are some narrower muscle fibers called intrafusal fibers as opposed to the muscle fibers outside the spindle called the extrafusal fibers. The spindles are attached to a muscle by their ends in such a way that when the muscle is stretched, the spindle is stretched. One end of a spindle may be attached to a tendon. Muscle spindles are involved in the stretch reflex or knee-jerk reflex.

Efferent Motor Nerve Fibers

Efferent nerve fibers are divided into somatic efferent and visceral efferent.

The cell body of somatic efferent fibers lies in the ventral gray matter of the spinal cord or in the motor nuclei of cranial nerves in the brain. Myelinated fibers form the ventral roots and the efferent fibers terminate in skeletal muscles of the body and head.

A muscle fiber and a motor neuron constitute a motor unit. Finer muscles concerned with precise movements have an abundant nerve supply such as the extrinsic muscles of the eye, which have a 1:1 ratio of neuron to muscle fiber. Motor units of other muscles may include up to 1:600 muscle fibers.

The nerve fibers will branch and terminate in a series of bulbous expansions at the motor end plates. The Schwann cell covering replaces the myelin as an axon sheath and covers the upper part of the axolemma. The lower part of the terminal axolemma rests in a groove of the sarcolemma called the synaptic gutter. The sarcolemma on the floor of the synaptic gutter has many junctional folds that increase the surface area and are separated from the sarcolemma by a 20 nm wide space called the synaptic cleft.

Postganglionic visceral efferent fibers from the autonomic ganglia terminate in heart muscle, smooth muscle of the viscera, and blood vessels and glandular epithelia.

Figure 7.1 Myelinated and nonmyelinated axon of peripheral nerve: Nu = nucleus of Schwann cell; My = myelin sheath; Ma = myelinated axon; NMa = nonmyelinated axon; Col = collagen.

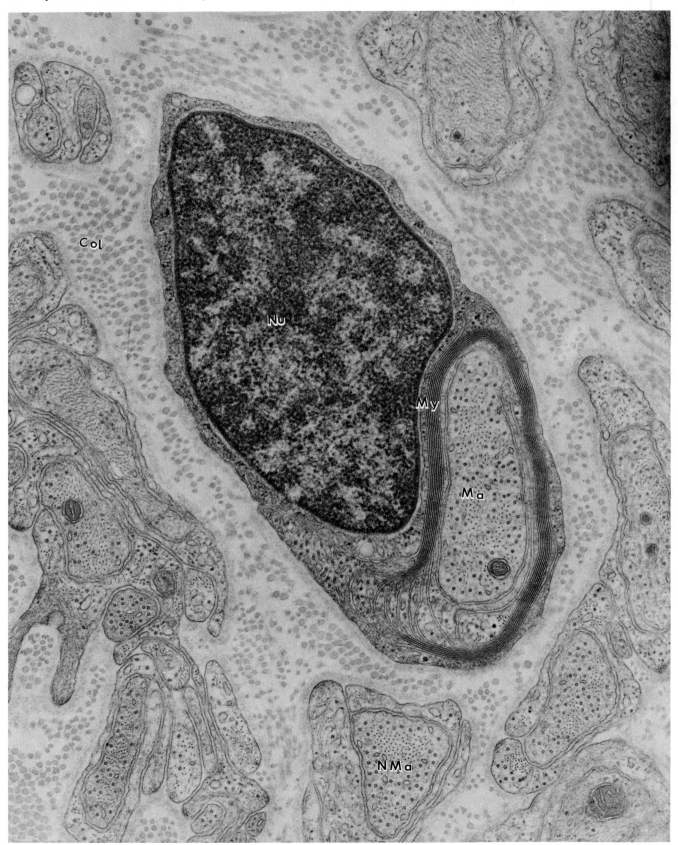

Neuroglia (Glia)

In addition to cells that transmit stimuli, the central nervous system contains many nontransmitting cells that are called neuroglia. They are essential for permitting the cell bodies and processes of neurons to be arranged and maintained in a proper spatial configuration with one another. Neuroglia are not stained by H&E but are stained by silver and gold impregnation techniques developed by Cajal and Golgi.

Neuroglia are divided into astroglia, oligodendria, microglia, and ependyma.

Astroglia

Astroglia are the most common neuroglia cells and contain branching and long slender processes. Astroglia are further divided into the *fibrous astrocytes,* which contain long slender processes and are located in the white matter, and *protoplasmic astrocytes,* which are thicker and contain many branch processes and are located in the gray matter of the brain and spinal cord. The processes are in close contact with walls of blood vessels of the nervous system by structures called *sucker feet.* Astrocytes play a role in scar formation in the CNS when they react to injury and proliferate to form scar tissue by a process called *gliosis.*

Oligodendria

Oligodendria have short, beaded processes, smaller and darker nuclei compared to those of other neuroglia cells, and a dense cytoplasm containing ribosomes, mitochondria, and microtubules. Oligodendria may be *perivascular* when they are adjacent to blood vessels, *perineuronal* when they are adjacent to neuron cell bodies, or *interfascicular* when they are found in white matter. Their wide flattened processes wrap around nerve fibers in successive layers that become converted into myelin.

Microglia

Microglia are the smallest of neuroglia cells and are mesodermal in origin. They have an irregular shape with delicate and tortuous cytoplasmic processes with delicate spines and show a deeply stained nucleus in silver preparations. These cells are phagocytic and may be part of the macrophage system. Microglia cells are found near blood vessels and throughout the gray and white matter. They become enlarged at cellular injury and phagocytose cellular debris by clearing necrotic tissue prior to gliosis.

Ependyma

The *ependyma* is composed of a layer of cuboidal or low columnar cells that line the cavities of the spinal cord and brain. In the embryo the cells are ciliated and contain microvilli; however, only a few ependymal cells in the adult possess cilia. The cells are closely packed with elongated nuclei and their long axes are perpendicular to the cavity of the spinal cord. In the ventricles of the brain, the ependyma is modified to form the special secretory epithelium of the choroid plexuses giving rise to cerebrospinal fluid.

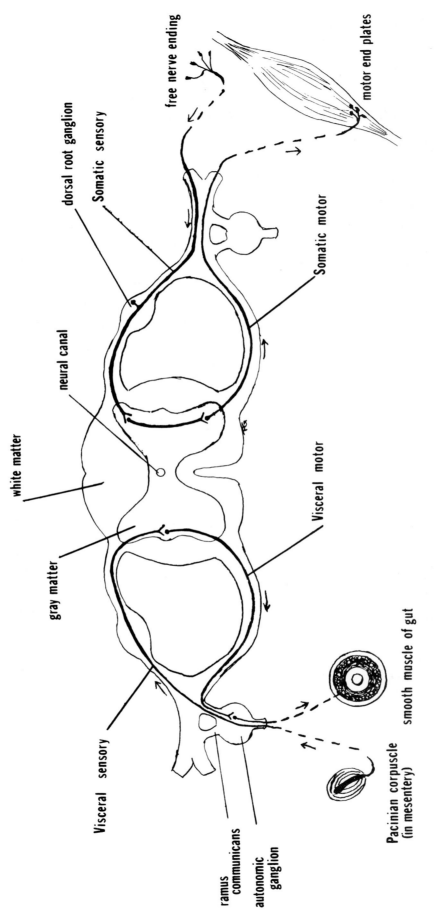

free nerve ending

motor end plates

dorsal root ganglion

Somatic sensory

neural canal

Somatic motor

white matter

gray matter

Visceral motor

Visceral sensory

ramus communicans

autonomic ganglion

Pacinian corpuscle
(in mesentery)

smooth muscle of gut

Spinal Cord and Autoomic Nervous System

Neuron and Sensory Organs

Label illustrations using terms listed below.

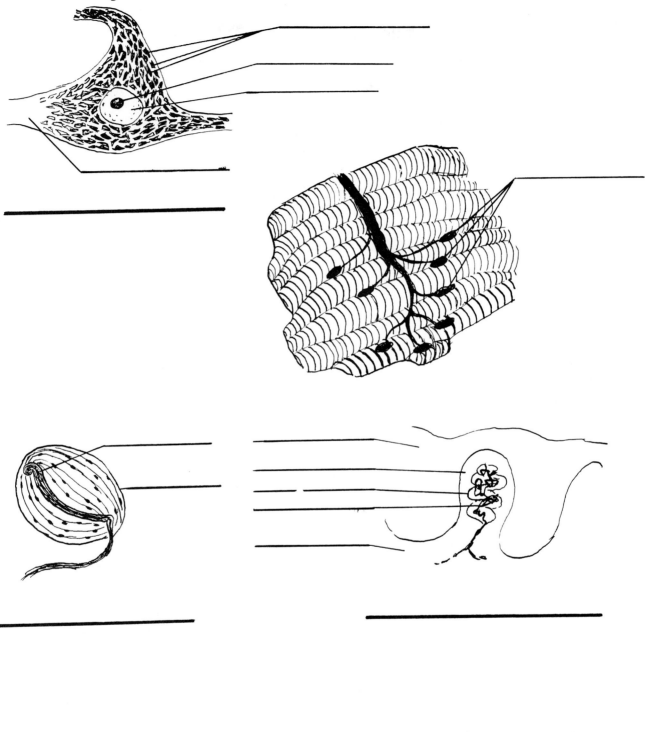

Meissner's corpuscle

capsule
dermal papilla
dermis
epidermis
nerve endings

Motor end plates
Pacinian corpuscle

capsule
nerve fiber

Neuron

axon hillock
Nissl bodies
nucleolus
nucleus

Slides

Examine the following nervous tissue slides and make drawings in spaces provided:

1. Nissl bodies, neuron
2. Nerve, mammal, l.s. & c.s.
3. Spinal cord—silver, c.s.
4. Spinal cord ganglion, c.s.
5. Pacinian corpuscle, w.m.
6. Skin corpuscle, Meissner section

Supply the following labels for each drawing:

1. Nissl bodies: nucleus, nucleolus, perikaryon, dendrite, axon hillock, neuroglia
2. Nerve, mammal: axon, myelin sheath, endoneurium fascicle, perineurium, epineurium
3. Spinal cord (a) (40x) anterior median fissure, neurocoel, white matter, gray matter, anterior horn; posterior horn; (b) (oil) anterior horn motor neurons, dendrites, nuclei, nucleoli, Nissl bodies, neuroglia, ependymal cells
4. Spinal cord ganglion (dorsal root): (440x) neuron, satellite cells, nerve fibers
5. Pacinian corpuscle: (40x) connective tissue lamellae, inner bulb, axis cylinder, nerve fibers
6. Skin corpuscle, Meissner: horizontal lamellae, connective tissue corpuscle, myelinated nerve fibers, naked axon

Draw the following tissue.

Nissl bodies (neuron)

Nerve (mammal) (l.s.)

Nerve (mammal) (c.s.)

Spinal cord (40x) (c.s.)

Spinal cord (oil) (c.s.)

Spinal cord ganglion

Pacinian corpuscle

Meissner corpuscle

Questions: Nervous Tissue

1. Cranial nerves are part of the _____ nervous system, whereas the spinal cord is part of the _____ nervous system.

2. Unipolar neurons are typically found in _____, and bipolar neurons are found in _____.

3. Nissl bodies of neurons structurally represent _____ _____ and _____.

4. A single bundle of nerve fibers within connective tissue is called _____.

5. The axoplasm of an axon contains numerous _____.

6. Covering the myelin sheath of internodal areas is _____ _____.

7. Afferent (sensory) nerve fibers are divided into two types, the _____ and the _____.

8. A connective tissue sheath enclosing an entire nerve is the _____.

9. A synaptic cleft is about _____ wide and contains the chemical mediators the _____.

10. A typical encapsulated lamellar sensory ending is _____ _____.

11. Neuroglial cells giving rise to cerebrospinal fluid are _____.

12. The embryological origin of microglia is _____ whereas that of astrocytes is _____.

Chapter 8

Circulatory System

The circulatory or vascular system enables blood and lymph to be distributed throughout the body. The system includes the blood vessels, heart, and lymphatics. The characteristics of the system are

1. a closed system of tubes through which blood is forced by the pumping action of a contractile heart
2. the presence of tubular walls that are permeable and enable exchange of materials with the environment such as tissue spaces and cells
3. a lymphatic system collecting fluids, colloids, and crystalloids from the tissue spaces and returning them to the blood stream
4. elimination of materials by transport to the kidneys, lungs, and skin

   Blood vessels are divided into capillaries, arteries, and veins.

Capillaries

Capillaries are very numerous and delicate tubes that anastomose and have a diameter of 7–9 μm. The total cross-sectional area of the capillary bed is very great, causing the blood to flow under low pressure. The walls are made up of one coat of simple squamous epithelium, which is an endothelium lining on a basement membrane.

There are two types of capillaries: continuous capillaries (muscle capillaries) and fenestrated capillaries (visceral capillaries). The external surfaces of the cells lining the capillaries rest on a basal lamina that is a product mainly of epithelial origin and their walls are held together by cell junctions of the zona occludens type. In the continuous capillaries, tissue fluid will enter or leave between the borders of the contiguous endothelial cells. There are spaces between sites where the outer lamina of the cell membranes of continuous endothelial cells are used. These intracellular spaces hold back protein but not water and simple solutions. Macromolecules may pass through by pinocytotic vesicles. The fenestrated, or perforated, capillaries are characterized by the presence of pores in the walls of the endothelial cells. These pores are often closed by a diaphragm that is thinner than the cell membrane. Fenestrated capillaries are usually found in tissues where a rapid interchange of substances occurs between the tissues and the blood such as in the intestinal villi and glomerular capillaries of the kidney (fig. 8.1).

Arteriole capillaries adjacent to arterioles are encircled by muscles referred to as precapillary sphincters, which are innervated by postganglionic sympathetic nerve fibers. Contraction of the precapillary sphincters permits the control of the amount of blood entering the capillary bed. After leaving the metarteriole region of the capillary bed, the capillaries branch into a central channel (thoroughfare channel) before reaching the venous capillaries and the venule.

Arteries

Blood is carried from the heart to the capillaries by arteries. There are three types of arteries, (1) elastic, (2) muscular (distributing arteries), and (3) arterioles.

The elastic arteries such as the aorta are large and contain many layers of elastic fibers that enable arterial pressure during and between ventricular contractions to be maintained. The muscular, or distribution, arteries are medium-sized arteries that can respond to nervous stimuli and regulate the size of lumen, thus controlling the flow of blood. The arterioles are small arteries with a narrow lumen and thin muscular walls. Blood pressure in the arterioles is maintained by the autonomic nervous system and hormonal control of the tonus of the smooth muscles surrounding the arterioles.

There are three tissue layers in arteries:

1. Tunica intima (innermost), which is composed of (a) an inner endothelial lining on a basement membrane; (b) subendothial connective tissue, and (c) internal elastic lamina
2. Tunica media, which is composed of (a) smooth muscle cells (spiraling or circular) and (b) reticular and elastic fibers

Figure 8.1 Muscle capillary: Mus = muscle; Tj = tight junction; En = endothelium; Lu = capillary lumen; Nu = endothelial cell nucleus; Cl = collagen; ZL = Z line.

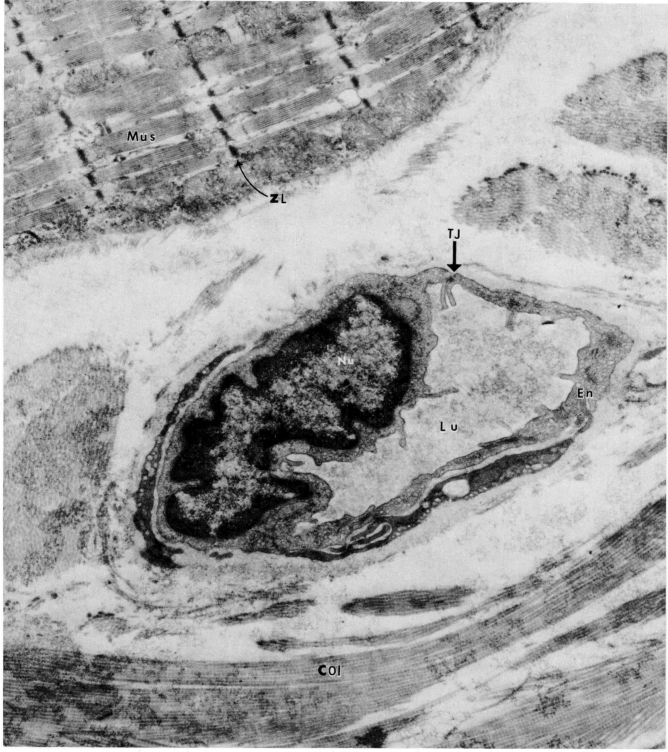

Muscle Capillary

Mus—muscle
Tj—tight junction
En—endothelium
Lu—capillary lumen
Nu—nucleus
Col—collagen

3. *Tunica adventitia* (outermost) composed of (a) external elastic lamina and (b) collagenous (white) and elastic connective tissue.

Small blood vessels called the *vasa vasorum* are found in the adventitia and outer tunica media, especially in larger arteries. These blood vessels supply nutrients to the arteries. In addition, lymphatic vessels are seen in the adventitia.

Small arteries, or arterioles, connect capillaries to muscular or distributing arteries. Small precapillary or transitional arterioles, or metarterioles, containing precapillary sphincter (smooth) muscles connect capillaries to arterioles. Precapillary muscles at the arterioles and capillary regions are regulated by the autonomic nervous system and by vasoconstriction and vasodilation, which regulate the blood pressure. Arterioles contain three to four layers of muscle cells when they are about 130 μm in diameter, and they reach a diameter of 300 μm before they are recognized as medium-sized arteries.

Muscular, or *medium-sized, arteries* are identified by gross dissection, possess thick muscular walls, and distribute blood to various organs. The elastic membrane of the intima often shows longitudinal folds (corrugations) due to postmortem contraction of the smooth muscle fibers of the blood vessels. The tunica media is the thickest of the three coats due to the large number of circular muscle fibers.

Large elastic, or *conducting, arteries* are easily identified by gross dissection and conduct blood from the heart to the medium-sized arteries. These arteries contain many layers of elastin in the intima and media that impart the resilience necessary to withstand systolic and diastolic pressure.

Veins

Blood is carried from capillaries to the heart by the *veins.* Veins have less collagenous connective tissue and fewer muscle and elastic fibers than arteries. They are collapsed when empty and also contain valves to prevent the backflow of blood.

Comparison of Arteries and Veins

Artery
1. Firm walls
2. Thick walls
3. Intima crinkled
4. Three distinctive layers*
5. Media prominent

Vein
1. Collapsed when empty
2. Thin walls
3. Intima smooth
4. Three indistinct layers*
5. Adventitia prominent

*intima, media, adventitia

There are three types of veins; small, medium-sized, and large.

Small veins connect capillaries to medium-sized veins. The smallest veins, or venules, are endothelial tubes surrounded by collagenous fibers and a few fibroblasts. Muscle fibers appear in vessels 40 – 50 μm in diameter and the adventitia become prominent in vessels 0.2–0.3 mm thick.

Medium-sized veins include practically all anatomically named veins and, except the main trunks, have a diameter of 1–9 mm. The *intima* is thin, containing a subendothelium with collagenous and elastic fibers. The *media* consists of small bundles of smooth muscle fibers interspersed with collagenous and elastic fibers. The media is especially thick in the veins of the lower extremities. The *adventitia* is well developed and consists of collagenous and elastic fibers often including bundles of longitudinal muscle fibers.

Large veins consist of a small intima containing an endothelial lining and elastic fibers, a poorly developed media with a few muscle cells and abundant connective tissues, and a well-developed adventitia containing longitudinally arranged smooth muscle bundles interspersed with collagenous and elastic fibers. Small and medium-sized arteries, especially in the extremities, contain *valves* that consist of two semilunar intimal folds projecting into the lumen that prevent the backflow of blood.

Lymphatic vessels resemble blood capillaries and function to collect tissue fluid and return it to the general circulation. They begin blindly as lymphatic capillaries and contain funnel-shaped valves to prevent the backflow of lymph. Lymph draining the intestinal villi and the intercellular areas will flow to the *thoracic duct* draining the abdomen, posterior extremities and gut, left thoracic region, left arm, left side of the head, and emptying into the left subclavian vein. The right side of the thorax and head including the right arm drain lymph into the right subclavian vein.

Lymphatic Organs (Nodules, Nodes, Thymus, and Spleen)

Lymphoid (lymphatic) tissue consists of reticular cells, fibers, and free cells, the *lymphocytes*. Reticular tissue is evenly distributed throughout lymphatic organs but lymphocytes may be concentrated into nodules or may be scattered as in diffuse lymphoid tissue.

Lymphatic nodules are dense, spherical aggregates of small lymphocytes lacking a connective tissue capsule. They may reach a diameter of about 1 mm. Nodules may be homogenous or may be organized into an outer dark cortex containing small lymphocytes and a light central area, the germinal center, which is sensitive to antigens and contains lymphoblasts and lymphocytes. Gut-associated lymphoid tissue (GALT) is represented by the tonsils, Peyer's patches in the ileum, and the appendix. The GALT is the source of B-lymphocytes in mammals.

Lymph nodes are oval or kidney-shaped structures reaching a length of about 20 mm. They are usually grouped in chains and are plentiful in the regions of the axilla, groin, and major blood vessels of the neck and mesentery. The indented region of the node is the hilum where blood vessels enter and leave. Nodes are covered by a capsule with the inner parenchyma having an outer cortex with nodules and an inner medulla with anastomizing cords containing B-lymphocytes and plasma cells. There are medullary sinuses between the cords and fibrous tissue trabeculae branching from the hilum and cortex. Afferent and efferent lymphatic vessels conduct lymph in and out of a lymph node.

The *thymus* is a triangular, bilobed lymphatic organ located superior to the sternum. It is relatively large at birth and begins to involute at puberty, which is related to adrenocortical and sex hormone secretions. The lobes contain a cortex in which are located small lymphocytes called *thymocytes*, which migrated to the thymus from the bone marrow and which give rise to T-lymphocytes. The less compact medulla has fewer thymocytes but more epithelial reticular cells. There is evidence that the epithelial reticular cells secrete the hormone *thymosin*, which appears to restore immunological competence to experimentally thymectomized animals. Also present in the medulla are acidophylic, spherical structures with concentrically arranged epithelial cells called *thymic (Hassall's) corpuscles*. Although the thymic corpuscles increase during thymocyte destruction and thymic involution, their functional significance is unknown.

The *spleen* is the largest of the lymphatic organs and functions to remove impurities from the blood by its phagocytic cells. In addition, it produces B-lymphocytes and stores erythrocytes. It is surrounded by a capsule and investing trabeculae both of which are composed of collagenous connective tissue, elastic fibers, and smooth muscle fibers. The capsule is covered by mesothelium. The *pulp* is supported by reticular fibers and is subdivided into white pulp, which surrounds the arteries in the central areas, and peripheral red pulp, which is infiltrated with circulating blood. The red pulp contains the venous sinuses, plasma cells, granular leucocytes, and erythrocytes.

The Heart

The *heart* is a large muscular organ that propels blood through the blood vessels and has four chambers. The wall of each chamber consists of three layers, (1) inner endocardium, (2) middle myocardium, and (3) outer epicardium.

The *endocardium* corresponds to the intima of veins and arteries with an endothelial lining of connective tissue, smooth muscles, and elastic fibers. The endocardium is a thin, glistening membrane covering the inner surface of the atria and ventricles. It is thick, especially in the left atrium, however, it is relatively thin in the ventricles and is continuous with the intima of the blood vessels.

The *myocardium* consists of cardiac muscle fibers arranged in layers and covering the heart chambers in a complex spiral manner. The myocardium is thin in the atria and thickest in the left ventricle. The muscle cells in this area are either contractile cells or conductive cells used for the rapid conduction of impulses. The special type of striated muscle tissue composing the myocardium also contains *intercalated discs*, which are observed as cross bands 0.5–1.0 μm thick, which represent specialized cell junctions with a complex pattern and with a variety of structural characteristics.

The *epicardium*, or visceral pericardium, is the serous membrane of the heart covered by an outer mesothelial sheet of single, flat or cuboidal cells supported by a loose subepicardial connective tissue layer consisting of elastic tissue plus veins, nerves, and nerve ganglia. Adipose tissue often accumulates in this layer.

The *pericardium*, or parietal layer, is a connective tissue membrane of fibers supporting the mesothelium. The pericardium faces the epicardium across a pericardial cavity, which contains a small amount of lubricating fluid that permits the heart to move freely during contraction and relaxation.

The *atrioventricular (AV) valves* (tricuspid or mitral) are attached at their bases to fibrous rings, the *annuli fibrosi*, which surround the AV orifices and in turn are continuous with the chordae tendinae. These valves consist of folds of endocardium covering a central region of collagenous fibers. Scattered smooth muscle fibers extend into the endocardium. The *semilunar valves* of the pulmonary artery and aorta resemble the AV valves except that they lack smooth muscle fibers, blood, and lymphatic capillaries.

The *impulse conducting system* of the heart consists of special muscle fibers regulating the succession of contractions. Elements of this system are the sinoatrial node; the AV node; the AV bundle, or bundle of His; and Purkinje fibers with reduced numbers of myofibrils, increased sarcoplasm due to glycogen accumulation, and larger and occasionally double nuclei.

Medium Artery and Vein

Label illustrations using terms listed below.

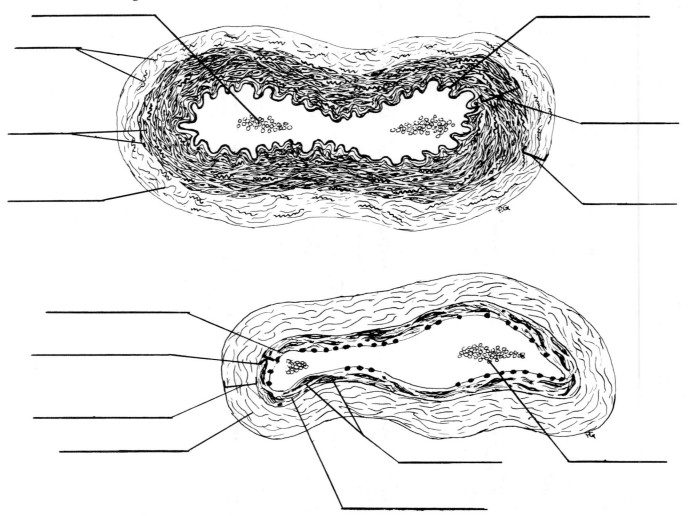

Artery

blood cells
tunica intima
tunica media
elastic fibers
muscle fibers
tunica adventitia
collagenous fibers
elastic fibers

Vein

blood cells
tunica intima
tunica media
muscle fibers
tunica adventitia
collagenous fibers

Lumph Node, Thymus, and Spleen

Label illustrations using terms listed below.

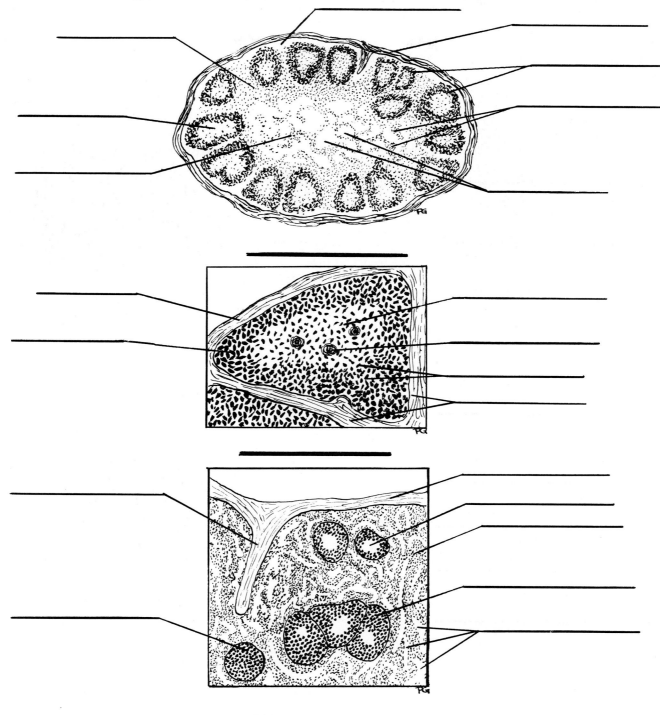

Lymph node	medullary sinuses	medulla	sinusoids
capsule	subcapsular space	septa	trabecula
cortex	Thymus	Spleen	white pulp
germinal center	capsule	capsule	
lymph nodules	cortex	germinal center	
medulla	Hassall's corpuscle	nodule	
medullary cords	lymphocytes	red pulp	

Slides

Examine the following circulatory system slides and make drawings in spaces provided:

1. Artery, vein and nerve, c.s.
2. Aorta, human, c.s.
3. Heart, mammal, atria and ventricles, l.s.
4. Spleen, c.s.
5. Thymus, c.s.
6. Lymph glands, c.s.

Supply the following labels for each drawing:

1. Artery: tunica intima (endothelium, basement membrane, subendothelial connective tissue, internal elastic membrane); tunica media (smooth muscle cells, reticular and elastic fibers), tunica adventitia (elastic lamina, collagenous tissue, elastic tissue). Vein: tunica intima, tunica media, tunica adventitia
2. Aorta: tunica intima (elastic fibers, smooth muscle); tunica media (elastic fibers, collagenous fibers, smooth muscle); tunica adventitia (collagenous fibers, adipose tissue, vasa vasorum)
3. Heart: atrium, ventricle, endocardium, myocardium, epicardium, Purkinje fibers
4. Spleen: peritoneum, capsule, trabecula, splenic pulp, venous sinuses, pulp cords, splenic nodule (Malpighian body), germinal center, lymphocyte
5. Thymus: capsule, cortex, Hassall's corpuscle, medulla, septa, lymphocytes
6. Lymph gland (node): capsule, cortex, medulla, nodules, germinal center, subcapsular sinus, lymphocytes

Draw the following from slides.

Artery, vein, nerve (c.s.)

Aorta—human (c.s.)

Heart—mammal (l.s.)

Spleen (c.s.)

Thymus (c.s.)

Lymph gland (c.s.)

Questions: Circulatory System

1. Two types of capillaries are _____ and _____.

2. A large elastic artery leaving the heart that dilates at left ventricular contractions is _____.

3. An arterial layer subject to the formation of cholesterol plaques is _____.

4. Small blood vessels that supply the adventitia and the media are the _____.

5. Contraction of precapillary sphincters will cause _____ _____.

6. Tunica adventitia is most prominent in _____.

7. Blood vessels that collapse when empty are _____.

8. The endocardium, which covers the internal surface of the heart, is homologous to the _____ of blood vessels.

9. The visceral pericardium is also known as the _____.

10. Large and occasionally binucleate fibers of the heart's impulse conducting system are _____.

11. Three examples of gut-associated lymphoid tissue (GALT) are _____, _____, and _____.

12. The part of a lymphatic nodule that is sensitive to antigens is _____.

13. Thymocytes arise from _____ and give rise to _____.

14. Thymosin is a hormone specifically secreted by _____ _____ cells.

15. The white pulp of the spleen surrounds _____ whereas the red pulp contains the _____ sinuses.

16. The spleen is covered by _____ composed of _____.

Chapter 9 Integument

The integument consists of the *skin,* the heaviest organ of the body (16% of total body weight), and associated structures such as *nails, hair,* and various glands. The skin is composed of an epithelial layer of ectodermal origin, the epidermis, and a connective tissue layer of mesodermal origin, the dermis, or corium. A subcutaneous connective tissue often containing many adipose cells (panniculus adiposus) binds the skin to the underlying organs.

The thickness of the skin will vary in different parts of the body depending on the relative thickness of the epidermis, dermis, or both. The interscapular region has thick dermis; the palms and soles have a thick epidermis and a relatively thick dermis.

The color of the skin is due to the presence of the pigments *melanin* and *carotene* and is also dependent upon the blood in the capillaries in the dermis and underlying connective tissue. The melanin is stored briefly in granules within the cells of the *stratum Malpighii* at the base of the epidermis. Melanin is formed from neural crest cells differentiating into melanoblasts and eventually into melanocytes with a formation of tyrosinase and melanin.

Although the number of melanocytes differs somewhat in the skin of the various human races, the difference in color is due chiefly to the manner in which the pigment is dispersed. In the Caucasian race, the melanin is found chiefly in the deepest portions of the Malpighian layer. The melanin provides protection against the action of ultraviolet rays, exemplified by a darkening of preexistent melanin and subsequent melanin release into keratinocytes plus an increase in the amount of pigment.

Epidermis

The epidermis is derived from embryonic ectoderm and consists of the following five layers seen from the dermis outward: (1) stratum germinativum; (2) stratum spinosum, the two previous layers identified as stratum Malpighii; (3) stratum granulosum; (4) stratum lucidum; and (5) stratum corneum.

The *stratum germinativum* consists of modified columnar or cuboidal cells with basophilic cytoplasm and oval nuclei containing one or more nucleoli. The cells rest on a basement membrane composed of a basal lamina and a reticular lamina. Desmosomes and hemidesmosomes on the inner cell surface facing the basal lamina are present. Many cells of this layer show mitotic activity resulting in the renewal of the human epidermis about every 12 to 14 days.

The *stratum spinosum* consists of cuboidal and polygonal cells (prickle cells) with a central and slightly flattened chromatic nucleus with a cytoplasm extending into spinous processes (formerly considered intercellular bridges), containing fibrils and terminating at desmosomes. The bundles of fibrils are called tonofibrils and are especially numerous at epidermal sites of friction, pressure, and abrasion where they maintain cell cohesion.

The *stratum Malpighii,* which consists of the stratum germinativum and the stratum spinosum contains melanocytes and *Langerhans' cells.* The Langerhans' cells are found primarily in the stratum spinosum and are star-shaped dendritic cells with an indented nucleus, and clear cytoplasm with some granules known as *Birbeck granules.* These cells are visible after gold chloride impregnation. Langerhans' cells arise from bone marrow precursors and have been recently reported to contain surface antigens common to most B- and some T-lymphocytes and monocytes. Recent evidence also suggests that the AIDS virus could lie dormant and reproduce in the Langerhans' cells before symptoms of the disease appear.

The *stratum granulosum* consists of two to five layers of flattened polygonal cells with central and oval nuclei and a basophilic cytoplasm containing keratohyaline granules, which are precursors of keratin, the major component of the cell type identified as a *keratinocyte.* The keratinocytes move upward in the epidermis as the keratin eventually replaces most of the cytoplasm and the cells flatten, die and are desquamated.

The *stratum lucidum* is a translucent layer containing thin, flattened, eosinophilic, nonnucleated cells. The cytoplasm contains a refractile material called *eleidin.* The stratum lucidum is readily observed in thick skin such as in the palms and soles.

The *stratum corneum* makes up the outermost layer of the epidermis and contains flattened, nonnucleated cells whose cytoplasm contains the protein keratin. The keratinized or horny cells at the surface are continuously shed or desquamated.

Dermis

The *dermis,* or *corium,* is derived from embryonic mesoderm and consists of two connective tissue layers, the outer papillary, or subepithelial, layer and the deeper reticular layer. Both contain collagenous and elastic fibers, with the deeper layer containing more fibers and fewer cells and with the papillary layer containing anchoring fibrils. Other components of the dermis are mast cells, fibroblasts, hair follicles, sweat (tubular) glands, sebaceous (oil) glands, nerves and sensory endings (Meissner and Pacinian corpuscles), smooth muscle fibers, fat cells, acid mucopolysaccharides, lymph vessels, and capillaries.

Hair and Glands

The *hair* is a thin, keratinized, epidermal structure with the lower hair root and the hair bulb within the dermis. At the base of the hair bulb is the dermal papilla. The hair is composed of three distinct layers, the medulla, cortex, and cuticle.

The *medulla* forms the central core and consists of two to three layers of large, vacuolated and moderately keratinized cells that are cuboidal at the lower portion but cornified and shrunken in the upper parts of the shaft. Intercellular spaces are filled with air.

The *cortex* surrounds the medulla, comprises a larger area, and consists of several layers of cuboidal cells in the lower portion and flattened cells at the higher levels. Pigment granules are found in and between the cells with air accumulating in the intercellular spaces modifying the hair color.

The *cuticle* is a thin, single layer of clear cells that are cuboidal midway up to the bulb, and farther up change from horizontal to vertical, flattened, heavy, keratinized, scalelike, nonnucleated cells.

The *hair follicle* consists of an inner and outer epithelial root sheath. The *inner root sheath* is composed of three layers: the cuticle of the sheath, followed by the middle Huxley's layer, and the outer Henle's layer. The cuticle layer has thin, scalelike overlapping cells; Huxley's layers consist of several rows of elongated cells whose protoplasm contains *trichohyalin* (eleidinlike) granules; Henle's layer has rectangular, slightly flattened, clear cells whose cytoplasm contains longitudinal horny, fibrils.

The *outer epithelial root sheath* is continuous with the epidermal Malpighian layer and demonstrates most layers of the epidermis. A connective tissue sheath derived from the dermis surrounds the outer root sheath.

The *arrector pili muscles* are smooth muscles bound obliquely to a special sheath of connective tissue and to the papillary layer of the dermis. Their contractions, stimulated by the sympathetic nervous system due to stimuli such as fear or cold, move the hair shaft into a more vertical position resulting in the so-called goose flesh.

Integumentary Glands

The skin contains two types of glands; sweat glands and sebaceous glands.

The *sweat glands* are simple, coiled, tubular glands distributed over most of the surface of the body while being most numerous in the palms and soles. The ducts do not divide, and the coiled, secretory portion is embedded in the dermis. Contraction of stellate-shaped *myoepithelial cells,* which surround the coiled portion, are responsible for discharging the secretion.

The secretory portion of the sweat glands is lined with a simple columnar epithelium resting on a basal lamina. Two cell types have been identified in the epithelium: (1) *dark cells,* resembling serous cells, with a broad luminal, surface and slender base, few mitochondria, abundant ribosomes, and secretory granules (containing glycoprotein), and (2) *clear cells,* pyramidal in shape, with no secretion granules, smooth ER, few ribosomes, and numerous mitochondria.

The *ducts* are lined with a double layer of cuboidal cells (stratified cuboidal) resting on a basement membrane. The cells in the inner layer are possibly involved in sodium resorption.

The typical sweat gland is of the *merocrine* type where the secretory granules leave the cell with no loss of cellular material (e.g., pancreas). However, certain sweat glands of the axillary, areolar, genital, and anal regions are of the *apocrine* type where the secretory product is discharged together with parts of the apical cytoplasm. These apocrine sweat glands are longer, open into hair follicles, and receive adrenergic nerve fibers. The merocrine *ceruminous glands* of the auditory (ear) canal and the glands of Moll in the margins of the eyelid are also apocrine sweat glands.

The *sebaceous glands* are usually associated with hair follicles and open through ducts (lined with stratified squamous epithelium) into spaces between the follicles and the hair shaft. The secretory portion consists of rounded masses or acinous cells. The peripheral cells are cuboidal and rest on a basement membrane, proliferate, and differentiate in the rounded central cells with many fat droplets and compressed nuclei. The oily secretory product, or *sebum,* is gradually moved to the surface along with remnants of dead cells. This is typical of a holocrine gland in which the product of secretion is shed with the whole cell, which involves the destruction of the secretion-filled cell. The secretory product contains lipids such as triglycerides, fatty acids, cholesterol, and its esters. The secretory process is controlled in men primarily by testosterone and in women by ovarian, adrenal, and androgenic hormones.

Skin

Label illustration using terms listed below.
insert line art from ms. page 168.

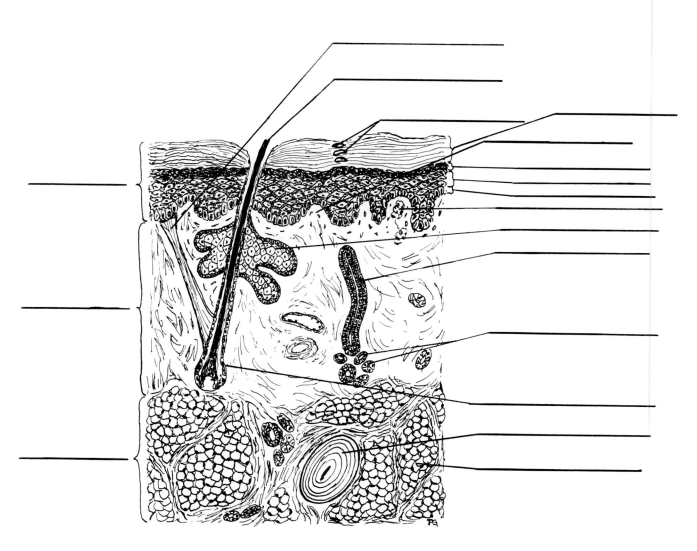

arrector pili (muscle)
dermal papilla
dermis
epidermis
fat cells
hair follicle
hair shaft
Meissner's corpuscle
Pacinian corpuscle
sweat gland duct (in dermis)

sebaceous gland
stratum corneum
stratum germinativum
stratum granulosum
stratum spinosum
subcutaneous layer
sweat gland
sweat gland duct (in stratum corneum)

Slides

Examine the following integumentary system slides and make drawings in spaces provided:

1. Skin: pig, c.s.
2. Scalp: human, c.s.

   Supply the following labels for each drawing:

1. Skin, pig: epidermis, stratum corneum, stratum germinativum, dermis, connective tissue, fibroblasts, smooth muscle, sebaceous gland, tubular gland, nerve ending
2. Scalp, human, c.s.: epidermis, dermis, connective tissue, smooth muscle sebaceous gland, hair follicle, papilla, hair shaft, hair cortex, hair medulla, root sheath

Draw the following from slides.

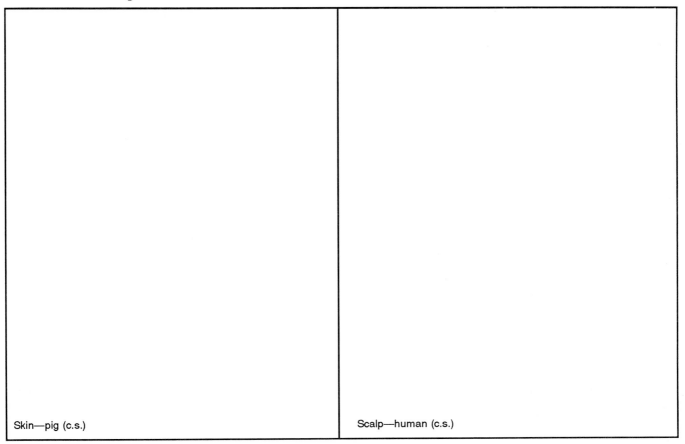

Skin—pig (c.s.)

Scalp—human (c.s.)

Questions: Integument

1. The generative layer of the epidermis is known as the _____.

2. The basement membrane is composed of _____ and _____.

3. The stratum germinativum and stratum spinosum are collectively known as _____.

4. Sweat glands and sebaceous glands are found in the _____.

5. In hair, pigment is usually found in the _____.

6. The arrector pili muscles are smooth muscles that move the hair shaft when stimulated by _____.

7. Sweat glands are tubular glands whose ducts are lined with _____ cells.

8. Sebaceous glands of the skin secrete a material known as _____.

9. The epidermis is derived from embryonic _____ and the dermis is derived from embryonic _____.

10. The _____ does not contain any blood capillaries or nerve fibers.

Chapter 10 Digestive System

The digestive system consists of the *digestive,* or *alimentary, tract,* which is a long, muscular tube that begins at the lips and ends at the anus. At these two sites the epithelial lining becomes continuous with the epidermis of the skin. The digestive system includes the oral cavity, consisting of the lips, cheeks, tongue, taste buds, and teeth; the esophagus, stomach, small and large intestine; and associated glands situated outside the digestive tube such as the salivary glands, liver, gallbladder, and pancreas.

The *lip* is composed of striated muscles of the orbicularis oris muscle. The outer covering has cornified stratified squamous epithelium containing hair follicles, sebaceous glands, sweat glands, and elastic fibroconnective tissue. The free margin of the lip has no hair follicles or glands and is relatively transparent due to a thick stratum lucidum. The epithelium of the free margin is richly supplied with blood vessels, which is responsible for the red color. On the oral surface, the lip is lined with a mucous membrane of stratified squamous nonkeratinized epithelium lying over connective tissue containing sensory nerve endings and the mucous labial glands.

The *cheek* is lined internally with stratified squamous nonkeratinized epithelium, which covers a mucous membrane, elastic fibroconnective tissue, and an inner layer of striated muscle.

The *tongue* is essentially a muscular organ composed of striated longitudinal, transverse and sagittal fibers arranged in interlacing groups and embedded in areolar and adipose tissue. The dorsal surface is covered by a mucosa modified to form numerous elevations, or papillae. There are three types of papillae:

1. *Filiform papillae* are the most numerous and are distributed in rows parallel to the V-shaped groove (sulcus) on the dorsal surface. They are conical in shape and covered by a keratinized epithelium.
2. *Fungiform papillae* are less numerous, club-shaped, and distributed singly among rows of filiform papillae. They are more numerous toward the tip of the tongue and they are covered by a thin, mostly nonkeratinized epithelium with a rich blood supply in the lamina propria and with taste buds in the epithelium.
3. *Circumvallate papillae* are the least numerous, 10 to 15 in number, largest of the papillae, and arranged along the sulcus terminalis. They are surrounded by a deep groove with walls containing large taste buds and a duct of deep serous or albuminous glands, *Ebner's glands.*

Taste buds appear as pale, barrel-shaped bodies arranged perpendicular to the free surface of the epithelium on the dorsal surface of the tongue and are associated with circumvallate and fungiform papillae. They contain an outer taste pore opening, the outer taste pore, and a small basal pit, the inner taste pore. The periphery of the taste bud contains supporting sustentacular cells and centrally located, columnar taste receptor cells, the neuroepithelial taste cells. There is a rapid cell turnover of the taste bud cells with average life span of about ten days.

Teeth have a dual embryological origin. Oral ectoderm will grow into the underlying mesodermal mesenchyme and will form the ameloblasts, which produce the enamel. The mesenchyme will give rise to odontoblasts that will form dentin. Teeth have a crown that projects above the gum, or gingiva, and a root embedded in the jaw. The tooth has a central pulp cavity filled with connective tissue that connects by a pulp canal and apical foramen at the base with the periodontal membrane. Surrounding the pulp cavity and forming the bulk of the tooth is the *dentin.* The dentin is a hard substance containing many inorganic salts and is composed of canal-shaped dentinal tubules running from the pulp cavity to the periphery of the dentin. The *enamel,* which is the hardest substance of the body, is composed of 97% inorganic materials such are hydroxyapatite. Enamel covers the crown of the tooth and contains enamel prisms formed by ameloblasts, which lay down enamel in concentric lines known as the lines of Retzius. New enamel cannot be added in adult life after the disappearance of the externally located ectodermal ameloblasts.

The digestive tract is composed of four histological layers: the mucosa, submucosa, muscularis, and adventitia or serosa.

The *mucosa,* which is the innermost layer, contains an epithelial lining bordering the lumen, a lamina propria containing areolar, or reticular connective tissue, and an outer muscularis mucosae.

The submucosa which is not present in the mouth or pharynx but extends from the esophagus to the anal canal, consists of areolar tissue with collagenous fibers in addition to glands, small blood vessels (Heller's plexus), and nerve fibers and ganglia (Meissner's plexus).

The outer *serosa*, or *adventitia*, consists of areolar connective tissue with nerves, blood vessels, and adipose tissue and an outer mesothelium covering, or serosa.

The *esophagus* contains the four histological layers of tissue typically seen in the digestive tract. The muscularis contains skeletal muscle in the upper fourth of its length followed by a gradual transition to smooth muscle in the lower portion. At the junction of the esophagus and stomach there is an abrupt change in the epithelial lining from stratified squamous to simple columnar epithelium.

The stomach contains folds on its surface called *rugae.* In addition, its surface has pitted recesses, the *gastric,* or *mucosal, pits.* The mucosa contains a tunica propria, which is composed of reticular or areolar tissue, in which the glands of the stomach such as the gastric, pyloric, and cardiac glands are located.

The *gastric glands* contain four types of cells: *chief cells,* which are low, columnar cells with the nucleus near the base and zymogen granules, which suggest the secretion of a glandular mucoprotein and the digestive enzyme pepsin; the *parietal cells,* which are relatively large, oval, or polygonal with central nuclei, and a fine granular acidophilic cytoplasm that secretes hydrochloric acid; *mucous neck cells,* which are relatively few in number, are cuboidal or low columnar containing an oval and basal nucleus with a fine, granular basophilic cytoplasm. These cells secrete mucigen, which protects the gastric glands from hydrochloric acid. *Argentaffin cells* are relatively infrequent and scattered between the basement membrane and the chief cells. Their cytoplasmic granules are stained black with silver nitrate. One type secretes serotonin, a vasoconstrictor causing smooth muscle contraction.

The *pyloric glands* are simple, branched, tubular glands composed of tall columnar cells with oval nuclei. The pyloric glands protect the mucosa from autodigestion.

The *cardiac glands* are so designated because of their location. They appear at the transition zone between the esophagus and stomach. Those near the esophagus have clear cells like the cells of pyloric glands whereas farther down the stomach lining parietal and chief cells appear.

The *small intestine* consists of the duodenum, jejunum, and ileum. Fingerlike projections called *villi* appear in the small intestine; between the villi are glandular pits referred to as *intestinal glands,* or crypts of Lieberkühn. Goblet cells are present. The first part of the duodenum is identified by the presence of Brunner's glands in the submucosa whereas the lower part of the ileum is characterized by clusters of lymphatic tissue known as Peyer's patches. At the base of the crypts of Lieberkühn are large cells with coarse granules that are chromophilic basally and acidophilic apically. These are the *cells of Paneth,* which probably secrete the enzyme lysozyme.

The *large intestine* consists of the colon, rectum, and anal canal. The inner lining is characterized by crescent-shaped semilunar folds. No villi are present in the large intestine. The mucosa contains simple, columnar epithelium, which functions primarily in the absorption of water. Goblet cells are present in addition to the crypts of Lieberkühn. The submucosa contains prominent and well-developed inner circular muscles and well-developed outer longitudinal muscles, which are important in peristalsis. The large intestine is covered by a serosa that is a thin, connective tissue layer covered by mesothelium that may contain large deposits of adipose tissue. Intestinal glands gradually disappear in the lower part of the rectum and the mucous membrane develops a series of longitudinal folds, the rectal columns of Morgagni. The muscularis mucosae also disappear, and about 2.5 cm above the anal orifice, the columnar epithelium abruptly changes to stratified squamous epithelium. The epithelium, which lies over the branched tubular circumanal glands, becomes keratinized in the region of the anus.

Digestive System

Label illustration using terms listed below.

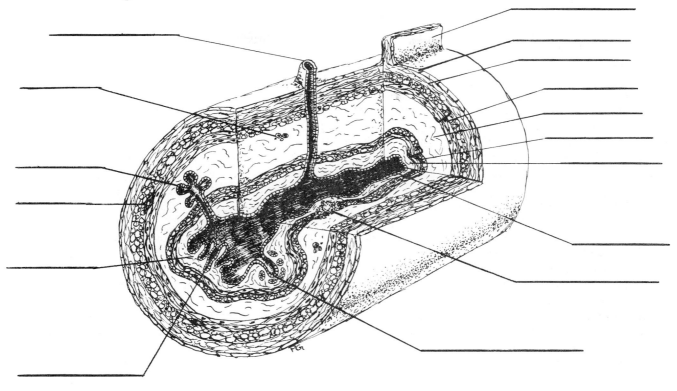

Auerbach's plexus	mucosa
crypt of Lieberkühn	mucosal gland
epithelium	muscularis externa
gland duct	serosa
lamina propria	serosal mesothelium
lymph node	submucosa
Meissner's plexus	submucosal gland
mesentery	villus

Fundus and glands

Label illustrations using terms listed below.

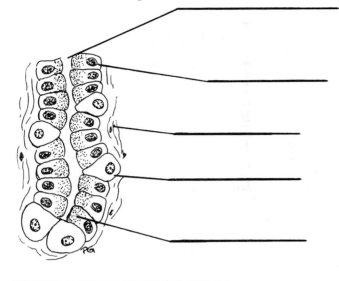

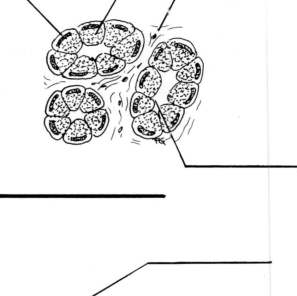

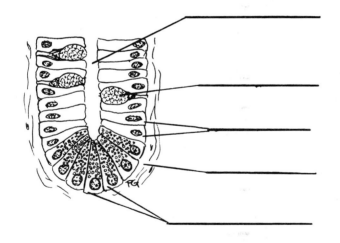

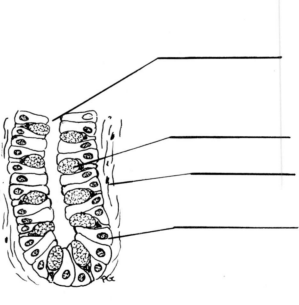

Fundus	*Glands (colon)*	*Glands (small intestine)*	*Glands (pyloric)*
chief cell	columnar cell	cells of Paneth	lamina propria
lamina propria	goblet cell	columnar cells	lumen
lumen	lamina propria	goblet cell	mucin
parietal cell	lumen	lamina propria	nucleus
zymogen granules		lumen	

Slides

Examine the following digestive system slides and make drawings in spaces provided:

1. Esophagus, c.s.
2. Esophagus—stomach junction, l.s.
3. Stomach—fundic, c.s.
4. Stomach—pyloric, c.s.
5. Duodenum, c.s.
6. Jejunum, c.s.
7. Ileum, c.s.
8. Peyer's patches, c.s.
9. Colon, c.s.
10. Rectoanal junction, l.s.

Supply the following labels for each drawing:

1. Esophagus: stratified squamous epithelium, striated muscle, smooth muscle, lamina propria, esophageal glands
2. Esophagus—stomach junction: stratified squamous epithelium, simple columnar epithelium
3. Stomach—fundic: gastric pits, fundic glands, mucous cells, parietal cell, chief cell, enterochromaffin (argentaffin) cell
4. Stomach—pyloric: pyloric glands, mucous secreting cells, parietal cells
5. Duodenum: villi, intestinal glands, duodenal glands
6. Jejunum: villi, intestinal glands
7. Ileum: villi, goblet cells, Paneth cells, enterochromaffin cells, capillaries, lacteals
8. Peyer's patches: lymphatic nodules, lamina propria
9. Colon: intestinal glands, goblet cells, lamina propria, muscularis mucosa
10. Rectoanal junction: columnar epithelium, stratified squamous epithelium, circumanal glands

Draw the following from slides.

Esophagus (c.s.)	Esophagus—stomach junction (l. s.)
Stomach—fundic (c.s.)	Stomach—pyloric (c.s.)

Duodenum (c.s.)

Jejunum (c.s.)

Ileum (c.s.)

Peyer's patches (c.s.)

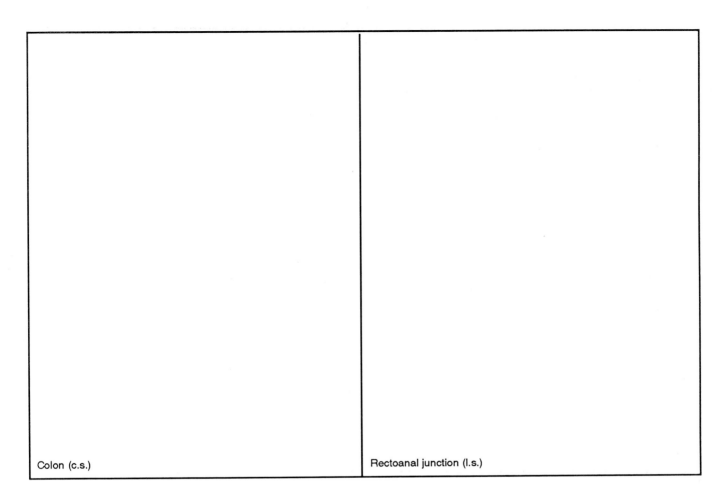

Colon (c.s.)

Rectoanal junction (l.s.)

Questions: Digestive System

1. The lip is covered with _____ _____ _____ epithelium.

2. The outer margin of the lip contains _____ follicles, _____, and _____ glands.

3. Three papillae of the tongue are _____, _____, and _____.

4. Taste buds contain _____ and _____ cells.

5. Embryologically, enamel is derived from _____ and dentin from _____.

6. The upper portion of the esophagus contains _____ muscle cells.

7. In the gastric glands, chief cells secrete _____ whereas parietal cells secrete _____.

8. Stratified squamous epithelium changes abruptly into simple columnar at _____ and also at _____.

9. The duodenum may be identified histologically by the presence of _____ glands.

10. Peyer's patches are typically found in the _____ and are known to produce _____.

11. Enzyme secreting cells at the base of the crypts of Lieberkühn are the _____.

12. The columns of Morgagni are found in _____.

Chapter 11
Glands Associated with the Digestive Tract

Large tubuloalveolar glands lying outside the limits of the digestive tube and pouring their secretions into the tract by ducts are the salivary glands, liver, pancreas and gallbladder.

The *salivary glands* consist of a glandular epithelium, the *parenchyma,* and a supporting interstitial connective tissue, the *stroma.* Connective tissue septa divide the glands into lobes and lobules. Collecting ducts, blood vessels, and nerve elements are located in the septa. The glands are composed of structural and functional units called the *adenomeres* containing a secretory portion of glandular cells (serous acinus or mucus acinus) and a conducting portion of intercalated or striated ducts. The glands are surrounded by a capsule of connective tissue containing collagen fibers.

The salivary glands are the parotid, submandibular (submaxillary), and sublingual.

The *parotid gland,* the largest salivary gland, is entirely serous in structure, has a complex duct system, and pours its secretion by the main excretory duct (Stensen's duct) into the oral cavity opposite the second upper molar tooth. The serous alveoli are located at the terminal portions of the intercalary, or striated, ducts and contain almost exclusively seromucous cells, which are periodic acid-Schiff (PAS) positive and with secretory granules rich in proteins showing a high amylase activity. The ducts are lined with simple columnar epithelium with cells containing central, spheroidal nuclei, acidophilic cytoplasm, and characteristic striations at the basal portion. It has been suggested that because of structural similarity between these cells and those of the distal convoluted tubules of the kidney, that they may also be involved in fluid resorption from the lumen of the interstitium.

The *submandibular (submaxillary) gland* is a mixed gland containing both serous and mucous alveoli. The main duct (Wharton's duct) opens into the oral cavity beneath the tongue and is lined with pseudostratified columnar epithelium. The *serous cells* are wedge-shaped with rounded central nuclei, mitochondria, Golgi, and endoplasmic reticulum appearing as parallel filaments and adjacent to the nuclei, and zymogen granules whose frequency is related to the degree of activity. The *mucous cells* are cuboidal, or low columnar, and are grouped around the lumen containing flattened, basal nuclei, and paler cytoplasm. The serous cells do not border the lumen of the alveolus and are arranged in the form of a cap outside the mucous cells often appearing in sections as crescent-shaped demilunes.

The *sublingual gland* is also a mixed gland, lacks intercalary ducts, and is the smallest of the salivary glands. The alveoli open directly into short secretory channels and have mucous cells bordering the lumen with large serous crescents or demilunes bordering the mucous cells. The gland does not have a distinct capsule, however, the connective tissue septa are well developed.

Liver

The *liver* is the largest gland of the body and has both exocrine and endocrine functions. The principle exocrine functions of the liver are the production of bile, prothrombin, serum albumin, and lipoproteins; the storage of carbohydrates (such as glycogen), proteins, fats, and vitamins; and the deamination, detoxification, and excretion of several compounds. The liver is divided into four lobes and is covered by a tunica serosa within which is a delicate connective tissue capsule, the *capsule of Glisson.* This capsule is composed of elastic fibers, covers the entire surface of the liver, and forms a continuous inner framework dividing the liver into many small lobules.

The *hepatic lobules* may be considered the anatomical units of structure of the liver, are roughly hexagonal, and contain a system of polyhedral cells arranged as hepatic cords, which are irregular, branching, interconnected plates. In addition, a system of anastamosing blood sinusoids is observed.

The *hepatic cords* appear to converge at a central vein in the middle of a lobule. Between the lobules are *portal canals,* which are roughly triangular in shape and contain branches of the hepatic artery, portal vein, and bile duct. Along the parallel sides of the lobules are interlobular veins.

The *hepatic sinusoids* are lined with endothelial cells containing small, dark nuclei with cytoplasm forming a thin film along the border of the sinusoid. In addition, large stellate, phagocytic cells with pale oval nuclei, pseudopodia, and microvilli are observed, which are called *Kupffer's cells.*

The *hepatic cells* (hepatocytes) are large, polyhedral cells with a large spheroidal nucleus that occasionally may be double. In addition, a prominent nucleolus is observed. The hepatic cells also contain mitochondria, Golgi apparatus, smooth and rough ER, granules containing glycogen, lipid and bile pigment, and lysosomes. Midway along the interface between adjacent hepatic cells are irregularly branching minute channels called the *bile canaliculi*. The hepatocytes transform and transport blood components into the bile canaliculi. The resulting bile containing bile acids, bilirubin, and water then flows from the bile canaliculi to the bile ductules and the bile ducts, eventually reaching the hepatic duct.

The Pancreas

The *pancreas* is a large gland in the abdomen with its head resting in the concavity of the duodenum and its body extending toward the spleen. In its embryonic development, it arises during the fourth week of gestation as two separate endodermal outpocketings of the developing duodenum (i.e., the dorsal pancreas and the ventral pancreas). The dorsal pancreas connects by an accessory duct (duct of Santorini) to the duodenum above the common bile duct whereas the ventral pancreas connects by its main duct (duct of Wirsung) to the common bile duct, which then empties into the duodenum. The two lobes of the pancreas join in later embryonic development, but the ducts remain separate.

The pancreas is enclosed by a thin, connective tissue capsule that separates the pancreas from adjacent structures and is covered with peritoneum. Partitions of connective tissue from the capsule forming septa divide the pancreas into lobules. The lobules contain the *acini,* which are composed of pyramidal cells spherically arranged around a central lumen, which extends to form a duct. The acini and their ducts are situated in the pancreas in a random fashion. The cells of the acini contain nuclei near the broad base. The nuclei contain nucleoli. The cytoplasm is basophilic, especially in the region between the nucleus and the base of the cell. In H&E preparations this region appears deep purple due to RNA.

Between the nucleus and the apical portion of the cells are *zymogen granules,* which give that region acidophilic characteristics. The zymogen granules represent the result of enzymatic activity and are the secretory vessels that bud off from the Golgi saccules containing proteins. This previous activity represents the exocrine function of the pancreas. The endocrine function of the pancreas is associated with isolated clusters of cells, the islets of Langerhans.

The *islets of Langerhans* contain more or less isolated masses of pale staining cells, arranged in the form of irregular and anastomosing cords as seen in H&E preparations. Between the cords are numerous blood capillaries and a few connective tissue fibers. The islets are surrounded by pancreatic acini, however, they do not secrete into tubules and their secretion is considered endocrine. Special staining techniques reveal that the islet cells consist of three types: *alpha cells* making up about 20% of the islet tissue secreting glucagon, a hyperglycemic agent that elevates blood sugar; *beta cells* that secrete insulin, a hypoglycemic hormone that decreases blood sugar; and *delta cells* that may be a variation of the alpha cells. The significance of the delta cells is not clearly understood.

The Gallbladder

The *gallbladder* is a hollow diverticulum of the bile duct attached obliquely to the lower surface of the liver, and is pear-shaped in appearance. It consists of a blind end known as the *fundus,* a body, and a neck, which continues into the cystic duct. The *spiral valve of Heister,* composed of folds in the mucosa, is located in the neck.

The four common layers of the digestive tract are not clearly differentiated in the gallbladder. The mucosa inner lining is composed of simple columnar epithelium with cells characterized by generally basal nuclei, many mitochondria, and microvilli borders in the apical region. The mucosa is primarily involved in water absorption, concentrating bile five to tenfold. The columnar epithelium contains extensive vascular plexuses and a few scattered smooth muscle cells from the muscularis. The epithelium invaginates near the cystic ducts into the lamina propria forming *tubuloacinar* glands, which have mucus-secreting cells responsible for the production of mucus in the bile.

The muscular layer is thin and irregular with interlacing bundles of smooth muscle fibers and bundles of longitudinal fibers traversing the length of the bladder.

The outer surface is composed of loose connective tissue of serosa covered by a mesothelium.

The gallbladder, by resorbing large quantities of water and mineral salts through its mucosal layer, concentrates and stores bile that is produced by the liver. Contractions of the smooth muscles of the gallbladder are induced by cholecystokinin, a hormone produced in the mucosa of the small intestine.

Salivary Gland

Label illustrations using terms listed below.

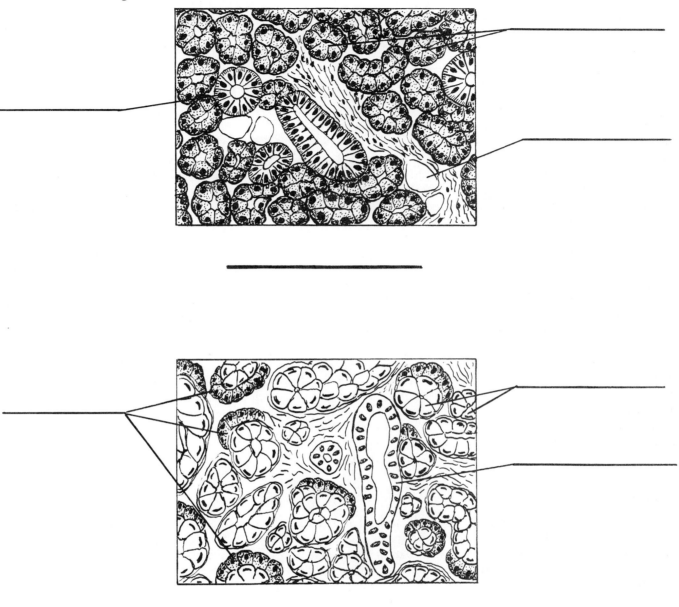

Mixed salivary gland
demilunes (serous cells)
excretory duct
mucous alveoli

Serous salivary gland
adipose tissue
serous alveoli
striated secretory duct

Liver and Pancreas

Label illustrations using terms listed below.

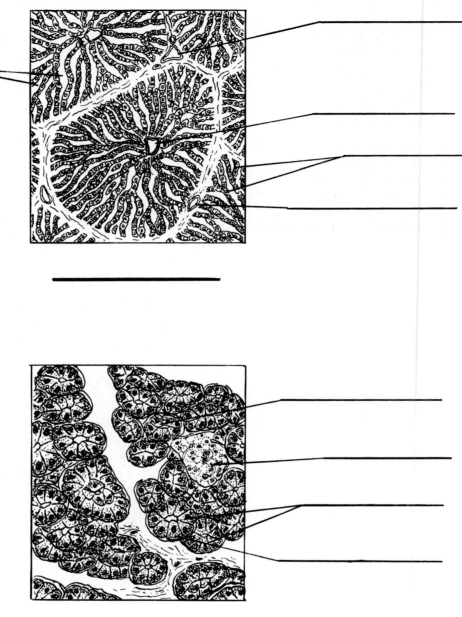

_____

_____

Liver
central vein
hepatic cords
interlobular vein
portal canal

Pancreas
acinar cell
acini
islet of Langerhans
zymogen granules

Slides

Examine the following slides of glands associated with the digestive system and make drawings in spaces provided:

1. Parotid gland, c.s.
2. Submandibular gland, c.s.
3. Sublingual gland, c.s.
4. Liver, c.s. (pig and human)
5. Pancreas, c.s.
6. Gallbladder, c.s.

Supply the following labels for each drawing:

1. Parotid gland: acini, seromucous cells, secretory granules
2. Submandibular gland: mucous cells, serous cells, demilune
3. Sublingual gland: mucous cells, serous cells, demilune, connective tissue septa
4. Liver: hepatic cords, central vein, interlobular vein, portal canal, bile canaliculi, bile duct
5. Pancreas: acini, acinar cell, zymogen granules, islet of Langerhans
6. Gallbladder: columnar epithelium, lamina propria, tubuloacinar gland

Draw the following from slides.

Salivary gland (parotid) (c.s.)	Salivary gland (submandibular)
Salivary gland (sublingual) (c.s.)	Liver (c.s.)

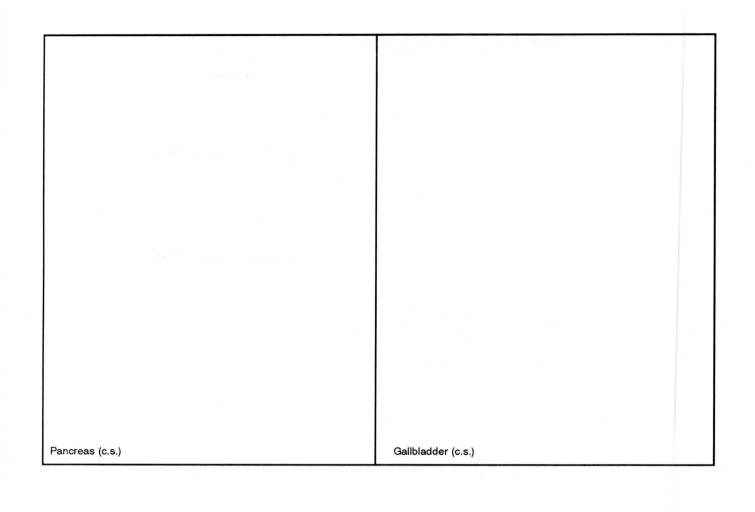

Pancreas (c.s.)

Gallbladder (c.s.)

Questions: Glands Associated with the Digestive Tract

1. The salivary glands are composed of structural and functional units called _____ .

2. The parotid gland is entirely _____ in structure, whereas the submaxillary and sublingual are _____ in structure.

3. Portal canals of the liver contain the two blood vessels _____ and _____ , in addition to a _____ duct.

4. Bile canaliculi transport their contents towards the _____ .

5. The hepatic cords appear to converge at a _____ .

6. Cells of the macrophage system found on the endothelial lining of the hepatic sinusoids are called _____ .

7. Pancreatic acinar cells have much rRNA because they are active in the formation of _____ .

8. The apical region of pancreatic acinar cells contains many _____ granules.

9. Pancreatic islet cells that secrete insulin are the _____ cells, whereas the cells that secrete glucagon are the _____ cells.

10. Epithelial cells of the mucosa lining of the gall bladder are typically of the _____ type.

Chapter 12 Respiratory System

The respiratory system is involved in the exchange of gases between the tissue fluids, plasma, and air spaces (alveoli) in the lungs. The air passing through the system must be filtered, moistened, and warmed to facilitate the exchange of gases. Mucus secreted by goblet cells entraps dust particles while cilia move these secretions to the oropharynx or the epiglottis.

The *vestibule* of the nasal cavity is behind the external *naris* (external nasal opening) and is the most anterior and dilated portion of the nasal cavity. The epithelium consists of nonkeratinized squamous epithelium with scattered sebaceous and sweat glands in addition to long and thick hairs called *vibrissae.* There is a lamina propria of dense connective tissue.

The *respiratory area* of the nasal cavity is the largest portion of the cavity and consists of a mucosa lined with ciliated, pseudostratified columnar epithelium with numerous goblet cells. Under the epithelium is a basal lamina resting on a fibrous lamina propria containing seromucous glands.

The lateral walls of the nasal cavities contain three *conchae.* These are bony expansions and in their lamina propria are venous plexi whose veins become swollen under conditions such as influenza or allergic reactions, thus hindering the free passage of air.

The *olfactory region* contains chemoreceptors in a specialized area of the mucous membrane in the root of the nasal cavity referred to as the *olfactory epithelium.* Three types of cells are formed in this epithelium: the *supporting cells* with broad, cylindrical apices, narrow bases, and microvilli on their free surfaces; the *basal cells,* which are small, spherical, cone-shaped cells of unknown function forming a single layer in the basal region; and the *olfactory cells* which function as bipolar neurons and are located between the basal cells and supporting cells. At their slightly dilated apex they contain six to eight nonmotile cilia that are sensitive to chemical stimuli.

The *nasopharynx* is the first part of the pharynx and is lined with ciliated, pseudostratified epithelium and in some transitional zones with stratified columnar epithelium. The underlying lamina propria contains mixed or seromucous glands. In the posterior portions such as in the *laryngopharynx,* lymphoid extensions appear as the pharyngeal tonsils or adenoids. In addition, the posterior wall is lined with nonkeratinized, stratified squamous epithelium. No submucosa is evident.

The *larynx* connects the pharynx to the trachea and its walls contain a series of fibroelastic connective tissue, which holds the larynx open at all times. The uppermost portion contains the *epiglottis,* which is lined with nonkeratinized stratified squamous epithelium with many seromucous glands in the epithelium. The mucous layer has two pairs of folds extending into the lumen: the upper vestibular folds or false vocal cords, and the lower or true vocal cords, which consist of two cords of elastic tissue controlled by intrinsic muscles of the larynx.

The *trachea,* which is continuous with the larynx and terminates at the bronchi, consists of 16 to 20 C-shaped rings of hyaline cartilage with the open ends in the dorsal aspect. The mucosa consists of ciliated pseudostratified epithelium with many goblet cells, a prominent basement membrane, and distinct lamina propria with elastic fibers and mucous glands. The submucosa contains areolar tissue, which lies over a perichondrium, hyaline cartilage, and muscle that corresponds to the muscularis of the digestive tract.

The *primary,* or *extrapulmonary, bronchi* resemble the trachea histologically with a gradual decrease in epithelial height in regions closer to the respiratory portion. The primary bronchi branch into three bronchi in the right lung and two in the left lung subsequently dividing into bronchioles and eventually terminating at the alveoli.

The *intrapulmonary bronchi* are characterized by smooth muscle completely encircling the epithelium and a lamina propria; numerous mucous and seromucous glands; and concentric and overlapping cartilage rings. The bronchioles lack glands and cartilage with the lumen lined by ciliated columnar epithelium with no goblet cells present. The lamina propria is then followed by an outer muscle layer, doubly innervated by the vagus nerve (whose stimulation causes constriction) and sympathetic nerve fibers (whose stimulation causes dilation).

The bronchioles lead into the *alveolar ducts,* which terminate in simple alveoli or in alveolar sacs. The alveolar ducts are long, winding and branching tubes with accumulations of collagen, elastic fibers, and smooth muscle cells between the openings of two or more alveoli or alveolar sacs. The epithelium consists of low cuboidal cells. The smooth muscle cells do not extend into the alveoli but the collagen and elastic fibers are present in the alveoli and alveolar sacs.

The walls of the alveoli consist of a thin, double epithelial partition common to two neighboring alveoli and called an *interalveolar wall,* or *septum.* The interalveolar wall is composed of three basic cell types: *endothelial cells* of the capillaries with nuclei smaller and slightly elongated as compared to the nuclei of the epithelial lining cells; *epithelial lining* of squamous cells, which fit together forming a continuous lining of the alveolar space; and *great alveolar cells,* or *septal cells,* which are cuboidal or rounded, are less numerous than the other two types, and generally occur at the junction of the walls of several alveoli. These great alveolar cells have large vesicular nuclei, abundant microvilli at their free surface, mitochondria, Golgi apparatus, well-developed ER, and characteristic multilamellar phospholipid containing cytoplasmic structures. The great alveolar cells secrete a phospholipid-containing substance called *surficant,* which aids in the lowering the surface tension at the fluid-air interface reducing the effort required for respiration.

The interalveolar septa contain macrophages also called *dust cells,* which are probably derived from monocytes. They phagocytose foreign particles, contain many lysosomes, and are passed into the alveolar lumen to be expelled into the pharynx. The septa also contain *alveolar pores,* which range from 10 to 15 µm in diameter and connect neighboring alveoli. They apparently function to provide intercommunication between alveoli thus equalizing pressure between alveoli.

Lungs

Label illustrations using terms listed below.

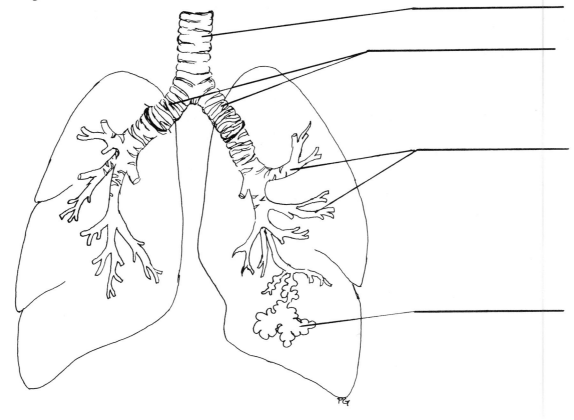

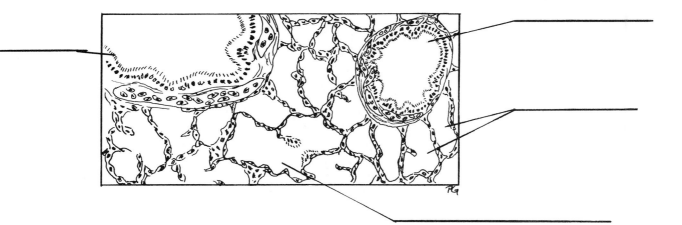

Lungs
alveoli
bronchi
bronchioles
trachea

Lung (c.s.)
alveoli
bronchus
respiratory bronchiole
small bronchus

Slides

Examine the following respiratory system slides and make drawings in spaces provided:

1. Nasopharynx, c.s.
2. Larynx, c.s.
3. Trachea, c.s.
4. Lung, c.s.

Supply the following labels for each drawing:

1. Nasopharynx: pseudostratified, ciliated, columnar epithelium, goblet cells, lymphatic tissue
2. Larynx: fibroelastic connective tissue, stratified, squamous epithelium
3. Trachea: pseudostratified, ciliated epithelium, goblet cells, lamina propria, hyaline cartilage
4. Lung: alveoli, bronchus, respiratory bronchiole, small bronchus, interalveolar septum, alveolar sac, endothelial cell

Draw the following from slides.

Nasopharynx (c.s.)

Larynx (c.s.)

Trachea (c.s.)

Lung (c.s.)

Questions: Respiratory System

1. The mucosa of the respiratory area of the nasal cavity contains _____ epithelium.

2. The nasopharynx is typically lined with _____ _____ epithelium.

3. Neurons of the olfactory epithelium are of the _____ type.

4. The cartilage of the trachea is of the _____ type.

5. The epithelium of the bronchioles is lined with _____ _____ cells.

6. The epithelial lining of the alveoli contains _____ _____ type cells.

7. Phagocytic cells in the interalveolar septa are _____ _____.

8. Two types of connective tissue in the alveolar ducts are _____ and _____.

Chapter 13 Urinary System

The urinary system consists of the kidneys, ureters, urinary bladder and urethra.

The *kidneys* collect metabolic wastes, especially nitrogenous products such as urea; regulate fluid balance of the body; produce *renin,* a proteolytic enzyme that stimulates the formation of the vasoconstrictor angiotensin; and also produce *erythropoietin,* a humoral factor stimulating the production of erythrocytes.

The kidneys are bean-shaped with an indented portion, or *hilus,* which contains the ureter, afferent and efferent nerves, blood, and lymph vessels in addition to three major and eight minor calyces, which unite to form the renal pelvis. The *renal cortex* of the kidney contains the capillary tuft, or glomerulus and the proximal and distal convoluted tubule of the nephron; whereas the inner area referred to as the *renal medulla* contains the loop of Henle and the collecting tubules.

The medulla contains 10 to 18 pyramidal structures, the *medullary* or *Malpighian pyramids* whose bases are in contact with the cortex with their apexes projecting into the minor calyces. These apexes comprise the *renal papillae,* which contain the 10 to 25 openings of the *collecting ducts.* The *medullary rays* containing straight collecting tubules continuous with the distal convoluted tubules penetrate the outer cortex. The loops of Henle connecting the proximal with the distal convoluting loops are located in the medulla.

The cortex contains Bowman's capsule enclosing the capillary tufts, or glomeruli, collectively referred to as the *renal* or *Malpighian corpuscles,* and the proximal and distal convoluted tubules. These structures, in addition to the loop of Henle, make up the excretory units of the kidney, the *nephrons.*

The *afferent* and *efferent arterioles* enter and leave the glomerulus at the vascular pole of the renal corpuscle. The entering arteriole divides into three to five large capillaries, which further divide into smaller branches eventually reuniting to form the efferent arteriole. Renal glomeruli close to the medulla are termed *juxtamedullary glomeruli.* The kidney receives blood from the renal artery, which branches into the interlobular arteries located between the conical-shaped Malpighian pyramids in the renal medulla. At the base of the pyramids, the interlobular arteries form the arcuate arteries, which lead along the corticomedullary junction. The interlobular arteries then branch off at right angles into the cortex. The afferent arterioles arising from the interlobular arteries lead into the afferent arterioles of the glomerulus where filtration takes place. Capillaries of the cortex collect at the stellate veins, which empty into the interlobular veins. The efferent arterioles lead from the glomeruli to supply the majority of other portions of the same nephron. Blood filtered through the glomeruli flows to the vasa recti veins, which lead into the arcuate veins draining into the interlobular veins, the renal, the vein at the hilum of the kidney, and finally into the inferior vena cava.

Bowman's capsule contains an inner, or *visceral,* layer covering the glomerulus and the outer *parietal layer.* Between the two layers of the capsule is the capsular, or urinary, space, which receives the liquid filtered through the capillary wall and the visceral capsular layer. The parietal layer is composed of a simple squamous epithelium on a basement or basal lamina. The visceral layer closely invests the capillaries and consists of basically stellate-shaped cells, the *podocytes.* The podocytes contain several major or primary processes extending toward the capillary loops, and from the primary processes extend numerous secondary footlike processes, or pedicels, that attach to the outer surface of the capillary basal lamina. The interdigitating pedicels comprise an extensive system of clefts called the *filtration slits,* or *slit pores,* between pedicels.

The *proximal convoluted tubule* is about 14 mm long with an outside diameter of 50–60 μm. It is highly convoluted as it leaves the capsule followed by a straight segment penetrating the medulla as Henle's loop. Cuboidal, or low columnar, cells with rounded nuclei, acidophilic cytoplasm, abundant elongated mitochondria, an apical brush border containing microvilli lining the tubules, and a PAS-positive basement membrane are seen around the proximal tubule.

A straight segment of proximal tubule is continuous with the thin descending segment of Henle's loop. This portion of the loop has a diameter of 10 – 15 μm and is lined with flattened squamous cells and weakly stained nuclei (H&E), which appear to protrude into the lumen. Henle's loop continues as a U-shaped structure with the descending loop becoming a thick, distal, ascending loop, which is about 9 mm in length and 30 μm in diameter. The distal loop is similar in structure to that of the distal convoluted tubule. The loop of Henle is mainly responsible for the formation of hypertonic urine. The descending portion is permeable, permitting the free passage of water and sodium (e.g., sodium enters and water leaves— since in the medulla, interstitial fluid is hypertonic). The ascending portion is impermeable to water resulting in a loss of sodium and leaving the filtrate hypotonic.

The thick portion of Henle's loop then penetrates the cortex, becomes tortuous, and becomes the distal convoluted tubule that is lined with simple cuboidal epithelium. These cells are less acidophilic, and have no brush borders or microvilli as compared to the cells of proximal tubules. The distal tubule is 4 –5 mm in length, 22–50 μm in diameter, and much less convoluted than the glomerular arteriole. Its cells become cylindrical with closely packed nuclei and Golgi apparatus at the basal portion. This region is called the *macula densa* and may relate to the transmission of information to the glomerulus about the composition of the fluid in the distal tubule. At the distal tubule, sodium is absorbed and potassium ions excreted under the influence of the hormone aldosterone.

The *collecting tubules* receive urine from the distal convoluted tubules. The collecting tubules leave the cortex where they have a diameter of about 40 μm, and pass into the medulla where the diameter increases to approximately 200 μm near the papillae. In this region they are referred to as the *papillary ducts of Bellini*. In the cortical regions the tubules are lined with cuboidal epithelium, which is gradually transformed into columnar epithelium in the medullary regions. The walls of the distal and collecting tubules are freely permeable to water and subject to the effects of the posterior lobe hormone ADH (antidiuretic hormone). ADH increases the permeability to water of the distal and collecting tubules resulting in water being resorbed and urine becoming hypertonic. In the absence of ADH, the tubule wall becomes impermeable to water and the urine remains hypotonic.

The *ureter* receives urine collected at the pelvis of the kidney. It is a thin duct, 25–30 cm in length, and terminates at the urinary bladder. The walls of the ureter consist of a mucosa, submucosa, muscularis, and adventitia. The mucosa is lined with *transitional epithelium,* resting on a *tunica propria* of reticular and areolar tissue. There is no muscularis mucosae. The submucosa consists of loose areolar tissue blending with the adjacent tissue often making the submucosa indistinct. The muscularis consists of an inner longitudinal and an outer circular muscle layer. The adventitia consists of loosely arranged connective tissue and many large blood vessels, some of which branch and penetrate the muscularis and eventually the mucosa as capillaries.

The walls of the *urinary bladder* are similar in structure to those of the ureter and are lined with transitional epithelium. However, the walls are thicker with the thickness varying according to the degree of distention of the organ.

The *urethra* carries urine from the bladder to the exterior. In the female it serves as a distinct outlet for urine from the bladder, whereas in the male, it also functions as the terminal portion of the ducts of the reproductive system.

The female urethra is about 4 cm long, lined with stratified columnar or pseudostratified epithelium at the proximal end and with stratified, squamous, muscularis epithelium at the distal end. The muscularis is reinforced by striated muscle at the orifice forming a urethral sphincter. Glandular outpocketings similar to the glands of Littre of the male are present.

The male urethra is about 15–20 cm in length and is divided into three portions: prostatic, membranous, and cavernous.

The prostatic portion is 3–4 cm long and is surrounded by the prostate gland. On the dorsal wall is a projection, the *colliculus seminalis,* at whose apex is a small opening of a blind tubule, the *prostatic utricle,* a remnant of the Müllerian duct. Lateral to the utricle are the openings of the ejaculating ducts, the terminal regions of the sperm ducts. The prostatic urethra is lined with transitional epithelium.

The *membranous urethra* is about 1 cm in length and is lined with pseudostratified columnar epithelium. The external sphincter muscle of the urethra is located in this region in addition to the bulbourethral glands. These bulbourethral glands secrete a mucuslike substance through ducts that lead to the cavernous urethra.

The cavernous portion of the male urethra is about 15 cm long and extends to the end of glans penis. The epithelial lining changes from stratified columnar or pseudostratified at the proximal end to stratified squamous at the distal end. This cavernous portion of the urethra is surrounded by the erectile tissue of the penis, the *corpus spongiosum.* Mucous glands, or glands of Littre, are found along the entire length of the urethra.

Kidney

Label the illustration using terms below.

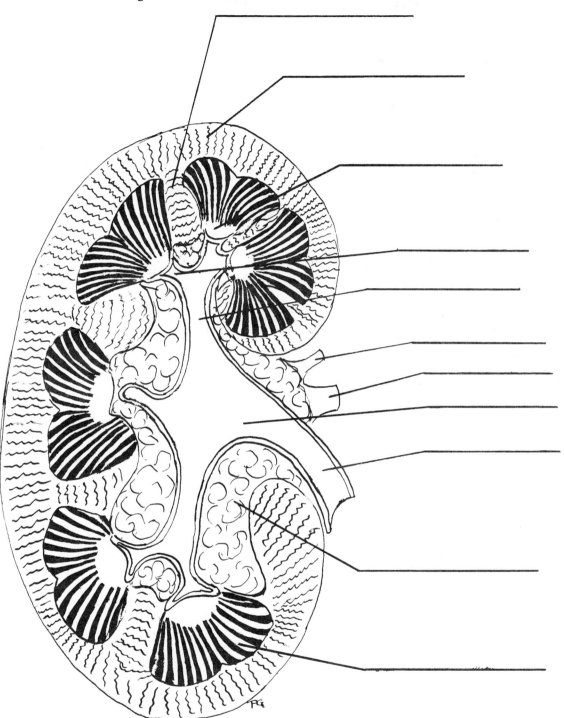

artery
cortex
fat (in renal sinus)
major calyx
minor calyx
papilla

pyramid (in medulla)
renal column
renal pelvis
ureter
vein

Kidney Tubules and Ureter

Label illustrations using terms listed below.

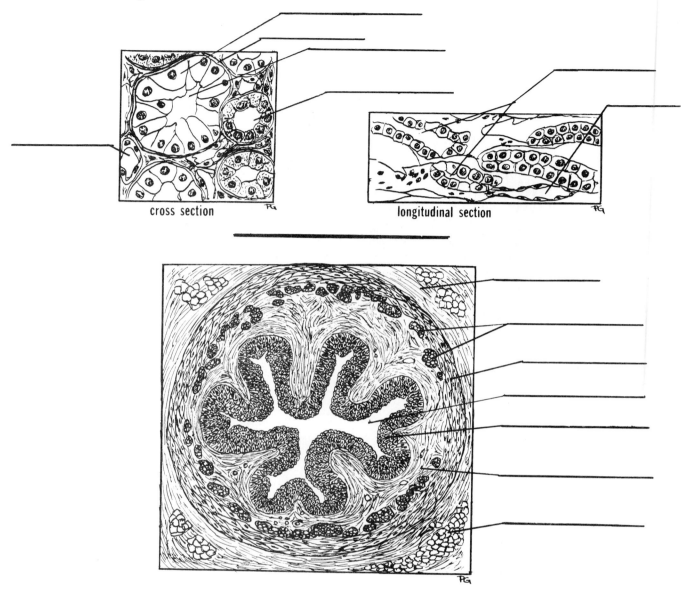

cross section

longitudinal section

Kidney tubules (c.s. and l.s.)

cross section:
  basal lamina
  collecting duct
  cuboidal epithelium
  thick section of Henle's loop
  thin section of Henle's loop
longitudinal section:
  collecting ducts
  thin section of Henle's loop

Ureter

adventitia
circular muscle
fat cells
lamina propria
longitudinal muscle
lumen
transitional epithelium

Nephron

Label illustration using terms below.

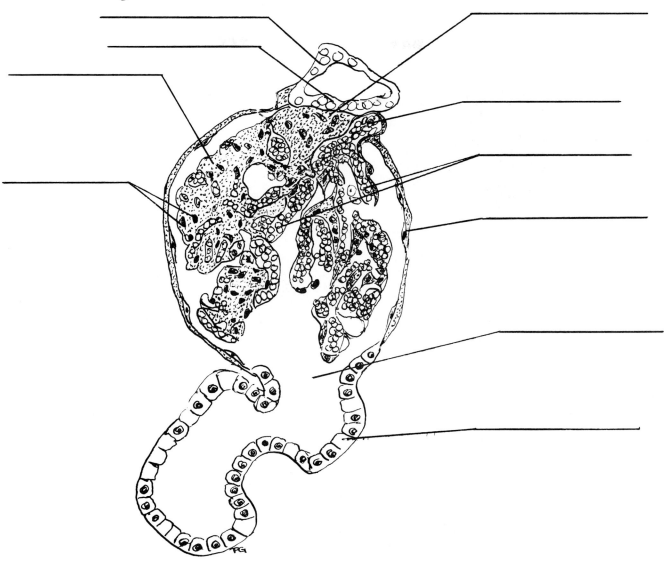

afferent arteriole
Bowman's capsule
distal convoluted tubule
glomerular capillaries
glomerulus

macula densa
nuclei of podocyte cells
proximal convoluted tubule
urinary pole
vascular pole

Urinary Bladder

Label illustration using terms listed below.

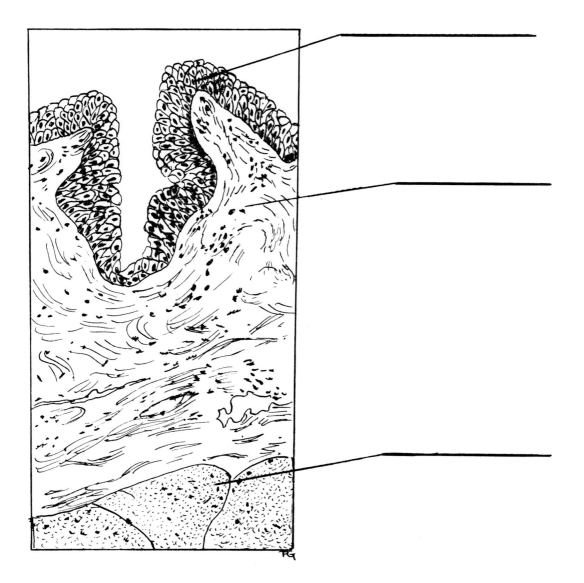

lamina propria
muscularis (smooth muscle)
transitional epithelium

Slides

Examine the following slides of the urinary system and make drawings in spaces provided:

1. Kidney, c.s.
2. Ureter, c.s.
3. Urinary bladder, c.s.

Supply the following labels for each drawing:

1. Kidney: glomerulus, capsule, tubule, cuboidal epithelium, interlobular artery, vascular pole of corpuscle, urinary pole of corpuscle, macula densa
2. Ureter: transitional epithelium, lamina propria, areolar tissue
3. Bladder: transitional epithelium, lamina propria

Draw the following from slides.

Kidney (c.s.)

Ureter (c.s.)

Urinary bladder (c.s.)

Questions: Urinary System

1. The parietal layer of Bowman's capsule is composed of _____ _____ epithelium.

2. The epithelium of the proximal tubule is composed of _____ cells, whereas the descending portion of Henle's loop has _____ cells.

3. The glomerulus and associated tubule constitute a structural and functional unit called _____.

4. The loops of Henle are located in the _____ portion of the kidney.

5. The visceral layer of Bowman's capsule contains stellate-shaped cells called _____.

6. Sodium loss occurs in the _____ of the kidney.

7. The walls of the distal and collecting tubule are subject to the effects of _____ hormone.

8. The mucosa of the ureter is lined with _____ epithelium.

9. A remnant of the Müellerian duct found on the dorsal wall of the prostate gland is _____.

10. Mucous glands found along the entire length of the male urethra are the _____.

Chapter 14 Reproductive System

Male Reproductive System

The reproductive system of the male consists of the testes, genital ducts, accessory glands such as the seminal vessels, prostate, and bulbourethral glands, and the penis.

The *testis* is a compound, tubular gland that has a reproductive and hormonal function. In addition, since it produces cellular elements, the spermatozoa, it is considered a cytogenic organ. The testis is surrounded by a dense fibrous capsule, the *tunica albuginea,* which thickens posteriorly as the mediastinum testis (corpus Highmori). About 250 pyramidal compartments separated by fibrous septa make up the *testicular lobules,* which in turn contain one to four seminiferous tubules embedded in loose connective tissue, blood vessels, and nerves.

The *seminiferous tubules* are convoluted tubules about 150 – 300 μm in diameter and about 30 – 70 centimeters long. Although some researchers believe that the tubules end blindly, others claim that there are intercommunicating arches between tubules of adjacent lobules. The tubules lead into the mediastinum, which leads into the rete testes, efferent ductules, ductus epididymis, ductus deferens, and finally into the urethra.

The walls of the seminiferous tubules consist of a capsule of tunica propria of fibrous connective tissue, a basal lamina, and a complex stratified epithelium, which contains the Sertoli cells and the spermatogenic cells with about five layers of cells each representing a different stage in the development of spermatozoa. The fibrous layer contains myoid cells with characteristics of smooth muscle cells, which in some species by their contractions assist in the transport of sperm.

The spermatogenic cells represent the various stages in sperm development, or spermatogenesis. Primitive germ cells, or *spermatogonia,* are clustered around the basal lamina. These cells are relatively small, contain the diploid number of chromosomes, and divide mitotically to give rise to primary spermatocytes, which marks the beginning of the maturation division, or meiosis.

The primary spermatocytes are relatively large cells (17–19 μm in diameter) and undergo the first meiotic division, which consists of prophase I, which in turn consists of leptotene, zygotene, pachytene, diplotene, and diakinesis stages; metaphase I; anaphase I; telophase I; and resulting in two smaller cells that enter an interphase stage at which time no DNA increase is seen. The cells then enter the second meiotic division, which consists of prophase II, metaphase II, anaphase II, and telophase II, resulting in small spermatids, which contain the haploid number of chromosomes and are situated at the luminal surface of the tubule.

The spermatids are transformed into motile spermatozoa by the process of spermiogenesis. The spermatozoa appear to be embedded in the apical portion of the Sertoli cells before they are released into the lumen of the tubule. Spermatogenesis occurs in a wavelike or cyclical fashion. The *spermatogenic cycle* is the series of maturation changes occurring in sequence between two successive appearances of the same cells along the same area of the same tubule. Each cycle in man lasts about 16 days and spermatogenesis ends after four cycles or about 64 days.

The *Sertoli cells,* or the nutritive (sustentacular) cells, are elongated pyramidal cells lying between the spermatogenic cells with their bases resting on the basal lamina of the seminiferous tubule and their apex extending into the lumen of the tubule. They have a clear cytoplasm and elongate nucleus with finely dispersed chromatin and one or more prominent nucleoli. The presence of lysosomes in the cytoplasm suggests phagocytic activity wherein detached cytoplasmic fragments from spermatids during spermatogenesis are digested. The lateral walls of the Sertoli cells have tight cell junctions forming the blood-testis barrier thus preventing the passage of macromolecules.

Pituitary follicle stimulating hormone (FSH) will stimulate the Sertoli cells to secrete an androgen-binding protein (ABP) that binds with testosterone secreted by the interstitial cells (Leydig) to stimulate spermatogenesis.

The spaces between the seminiferous tubules contain *intestinal tissue,* which in turn consists of connective tissue, nerves, blood vessels, fibroblasts, mast cells, macrophages, and interstitial cells of Leydig. The *Leydig cells* are oval or polygonal in shape with a large and usually central nucleus and with a granular eosinophilic cytoplasm containing peripheral vacuoles, lipochrome pigment granules, and crystalloids. Pituitary luteinizing hormone (LH) will stimulate the Leydig cells to secrete the male hormone testosterone, which is responsible for the development of male secondary sex characteristics. The Leydig cells arise from fibroblasts.

Mature *spermatozoa* within the lumen of the tubules are slender, motile, flagellated structures averaging 55–65 μm in length. They contain a head, which consists of a nucleus and acrosomal cap; a neck with a proximal centriole (at an angle about 45 degrees to the axis of the tail) and a striated connecting piece, which joins the nine outer dense fibers of the axial filament; a middle piece extending from the neck to the annulus (ring centriole) consisting of a filament (axoneme) of a pair of microtubules surrounded by nine outer doublet microtubules, nine course outer fibers, and a helical mitochondrial sheath; a principal piece, the longest portion of the tail, which consists of the 2 + 9 + 9 arrangement of microtubules and nine outer fibers and also a characteristic sheath of outer circumferential fibers; and the shorter end (5–10 μm) end piece of the tail consisting of two central microtubules surrounded by 9 microtubules after they have undergone the physiological process of capacitation in the female reproductive tract.

The genital ducts within the testis are straight tubules or tubuli recti, the rete testis, and the efferent ductules; whereas the extra testicular genital ducts are the epididymis, and the ductus deferens (sperm duct) leading to the urethra.

The transition between the seminiferous tubule and straight tubule is abrupt with spermatogenic cells disappearing first, then modified Sertoli cells disappearing abruptly, leaving a columnar epithelium, which is the characteristic lining of the straight tubules. The rete testis that follows is lined with cuboidal epithelium and the efferent ductules contain alternating groups of high columnar and cuboidal cells all of which are often ciliated impelling the spermatozoa towards the epididymis.

The epididymis is a highly convoluted duct, four to six meters in length, lined with pseudostratified columnar epithelium of rounded basal and columnar cells resting on a basal lamina. The apical region of these cells contains long, nonmotile cytoplasmic projections of microvilli, previously termed *stereocilia*. The functional characteristics of these cells are not completely understood; however, reabsorption and digestion of cytoplasmic fragments occur in addition to the spermatozoa becoming truly motile and fertile.

The *ductus* (vas) *deferens* is a continuation of the ductus epididymis. It has a narrow lumen and thick middle wall of spirally arranged smooth muscle fibers. The inner layer of mucosa consists of pseudostratified columnar epithelium with stereocilia. The outer lamina propria contains many elastic fibers. Before reaching the prostate gland, the ductus deferens dilates to form the *ampulla,* which has a labyrinthlike folded mucosa forming pocketlike recesses. The ductus deferens then narrows to form the thin *ejaculatory duct* (about one centimeter in length), which has simple columnar or psuedostratified epithelium but lacks a muscle layer. The ejaculatory duct penetrates the substance of the prostate gland and opens into the prostatic portion of the urethra.

The *seminal vesicles* are two highly convoluted tubes about 15 centimeters in length, which lie close to the ampulla and open into the ductus deferens at the junction of the ampulla and ejaculatory duct. The mucosa is folded in a complex manner forming many crypts. The epithelium is pseudostratified columnar with spherical basal cells. They contain cytoplasmic secretion granules and lipochrome pigment, which increases with age. The lamina propria has elastic fibers surrounded by a thin layer of smooth muscle innervated by sympathetic nerve fibers that surround the muscles to contract during ejaculation. The secretion of the seminal vesicles is alkaline and contains a globulin, ascorbic acid, and fructose, all of which are important in sperm motility and nutrition. The male sex hormone, testosterone, will proportionately affect the height of the epithelial cells of the seminal vesicles and the degree of activity of the secretory process.

The *prostate gland* surrounds the urethra and is an aggregate of 30 to 50 small compound tubuloalveolar glands with ducts emptying into the urethra. The gland is surrounded by a fibroelastic capsule containing smooth muscle cells. The capsule extends into the gland forming septa. The epithelium varies from columnar to cuboidal cells with some basal cells present. The nuclei are spherical and the cytoplasm contains secretion granules, lipid droplets, lysosomes, and shows intense acid phosphatase activity.

The individual glands of the prostate are arranged in three groupings: the inner mucosa glands, the central submucosal glands, and the outer main gland. Lamellar prostatic concretions, the *corpora amylacea,* occur normally in some of the alveoli. These are spherical bodies, about 250 μm in diameter, that contain protein and carbohydrate, increase in number with age, and may calcify forming calculi.

The *bulbourethral glands* (glands of Cowper) are paired structures each the size of a pea, located close to the bulb of the urethra and emptying into it. They are tubuloalveolar glands with columnar to cuboidal mucous-type epithelium. The connective tissue contains elastic, skeletal, and smooth muscle fibers. The nuclei of the epithelium are basally located, and the cytoplasm contains mucigen droplets and acidophilic, spindle-shaped inclusions. The secretion is clear, viscous, and mucoid.

The *penis* is a urogenital organ and is composed mainly of three cylinders of erectile tissue, the paired and dorsal corpora cavernosa, and the single and ventral corpus cavernosum urethrae (corpus spongiosum). The latter encloses the urethra. The corpora cavernosa are surrounded by a dense connective tissue of collagenous fibers, the tunica albuginea. The erectile tissue of the corpora consists of a network of spaces, or lacunae, lined by an endothelium of cavernous veins. There are a paired dorsal artery, a deep dorsal vein and a superficial dorsal vein. Parasympathetic nerve stimulation causes a relaxation of the smooth muscles of the capillaries and branches of the dorsal artery. Blood subsequently flows freely from the capillaries into the cavernous spaces enlarging the erectile tissue of the corpora cavernosa. The process is reversed by sympathetic stimulation of the capillary muscles leading to the venous drainage of the blood from the corpora cavernosa.

Female Reproductive System

The female reproductive system is composed of the ovaries, oviducts, or Fallopian tubes, uterus, vagina, and external genitalia. This system, which is controlled by hormonal and neural mechanisms is responsible for the production of ova, reception of spermatozoa, provision of a suitable environment for the fetus, expulsion of the fetus, nutrition of the newborn, and associated behavioral characteristics.

The *ovaries* are slightly flattened oval bodies about four centimeters in length, two centimeters in width, and one centimeter thick, each of which lies on either side of the uterus by the terminus of the oviducts. At birth the ovary contains about 400,000 follicles of which about 450 will mature and be released during the course of a woman's reproductive life. There are three types of follicles: the primordial follicles, the growing follicles, and the mature, or Graafian, follicles. The ovary consists of an inner medullary region containing blood vessels and loose connective tissue and an outer cortical region containing oocytes and follicles. A *germinal epithelium* of cuboidal cells covers the ovary. Under the germinal epithelium is a stroma of thick fibrous connective tissue called the *tunica albuginea.*

The *primordial follicles* are the only ones present before puberty. They consist of a primary oocyte, which is suspended in the diplotene stage of meiotic prophase and surrounded by a single layer of flattened follicular, or granulosa, cells. The majority of the oogonia have differentiated to primary oocytes by the fifth to sixth fetal month. The primary oocyte is a large cell about 40 μm in diameter with a large, eccentric nucleus, a large nucleolus, and finely dispersed chromatin.

The *growing follicle* consists of the primary and secondary follicles. As the primary follicle and its oocyte grow, the single layer of follicular cells forms the *zona granulosa,* which consists of cuboidal cells. An acellular, homogenous, acidophilic layer, the *zona pellucida,* develops between the oocyte and the granulosa cells.

The follicle grows into a secondary follicle primarily because of the increase of follicular cells and the accumulation of the serous fluid, liquor folliculi, within the follicular cavity, or antrum. The stalklike grouping of granulosa cells between the oocyte and zona pellucida is the *cumulus oophorus.*

The *mature, or Graafian, follicle* develops with the accumulation of follicular fluid. The granulosa cells become dislocated to the periphery of the antrum. The oocyte is surrounded by a circular cluster of granulosa cells, the *corona radiata,* which accompanies the oocyte after ovulation and is still present at the time of fertilization. Preceding ovulation, the oocyte along with the corona radiata detaches itself from the wall of the follicle and floats in the follicular fluid. A midcycle surge of luteinizing hormone (LH) from the pituitary precipitates ovulation, which is marked by the rupture of the follicle and the release of the oocyte. The oocyte passes to the oviduct and upon fertilization becomes an ovum, which begins division and is subsequently implanted in the walls of the uterus. Most follicles do not rupture or expel their oocytes at ovulation but involute and become atretic by a degenerative process leading to the death of the oocyte and removal of follicular remnants by macrophages. The follicle that matured and expelled its oocyte at ovulation gives rise to the *corpus luteum,* which will secrete the hormones progesterone and estrogen.

The follicular cells do not divide after ovulation but increase in size, assume the appearance of hormone secretory cells, and become the granulosa-lutein cells. These cells contain the pigment lipochrome in their cytoplasm, which is responsible for the yellow color of the corpus luteum. The cells of the theca interna give rise to the smaller and peripherally located theca lutein (paralutein) cells. Anterior pituitary luteinizing hormone (LH) will stimulate the formation of the corpus luteum. If pregnancy does not occur the levels of LH will drop resulting in the degeneration and disappearance of the corpus luteum, a drop in progesterone secretion, and commencing of menstruation. When pregnancy occurs, the placental hormone *chorionic gonadotropin,* which has LH activity, will stimulate and maintain the corpus luteum to secrete progesterone until the end of pregnancy.

The *oviduct* (Fallopian or uterine tube) is paired, about 12–15 cm long with one end opening into the peritoneal cavity to receive the oocytes and the other (proximal) end opening into the uterus. There are four rather indistinct regions of the oviduct starting at the ovarian end: the funnel-shaped infundibulum, the longer end dilated into the ampulla, the isthmus, and adjacent to the uterus the interstitial segment embedded in the uterine wall. The inner mucosa, lined with simple columnar epithelium with portions containing cilia that beat toward the uterus moving a viscous fluid along the other side toward the uterus, a smooth muscular layer, and an outer serosa composed of peritoneum.

The *uterus* is a thick-walled, pear-shaped structure with an upper dilated body, or corpus, with its rounded dome-shaped region, the fundus, and a lower cylindrical neck, or cervix, which opens into the vagina. The walls of the uterus consist of the inner endometrium, corresponding to the mucosa and submucosa; the myometrium, or muscularis; and the other serosa, or perimetrium.

The *endometrium* is lined with an epithelium of simple columnar cells with a mixture of ciliated and secretory cells. The lamina propria contains numerous tubular glands with deeper portions in the myometrium although they open at the surface. Anterior lobe pituitary hormones stimulate the ovary to secrete estrogen and progesterone that cause the endometrium to undergo the cyclic changes of the menstrual cycle.

The menstrual cycle consists of four phases the (1) *proliferative phase* (follicular), which follows the menstrual phase (day 1–4) and is characterized by the rapid regeneration of the endometrial wall, replacement of epithelial cells, and an increase in gland cells and vascularity (day 1–14); (2) *progestational (secretory, or luteal) phase* characterized by hypertrophy of endometrium, proliferation of glandular tissue, increase in edema and vascularity of mucosa (day 14–26); (3) *premenstrual phase* (day 26–28) is marked by constriction of the coiled arteries resulting in anoxia and anemia of the tissues, gland fragmentation, beginning of endometrial breakdown, and occurrence of blood and desquamated tissue in the uterine lumen; (4) *menstrual phase* (day 1–4) with endometrial desquamation, rupture of blood vessels, and bleeding.

The *myometrium* is the thickest tissue layer of the uterus and is composed of bundles of smooth muscle fiber separated by connective tissue. The interstitial tissue contains numerous large blood vessels, especially veins. During pregnancy, the muscle of the uterus is greatly increased.

The walls of the *vagina* consist of a mucosa, a muscularis, and a fibrous layer. The mucosa has transverse folds, or *rugae,* and is lined with stratified squamous epithelium with cells containing keratohyaline. Estrogen stimulates the vaginal epithelium to synthesize glycogen, which is converted to lactic acid by bacterial action resulting in lowering the pH of the vaginal tract during the estrogen phase of the cycle. In humans the surface cells are desquamated continuously. Although the epithelium varies little during the cycle, the condition of the desquamated cells is useful in the diagnosis of atrophic conditions and in the evaluation of estrogen therapy. The epithelium lacks glands but is lubricated by cervical mucus.

Graafian Follicle and Testis

Label illustrations using terms listed below.

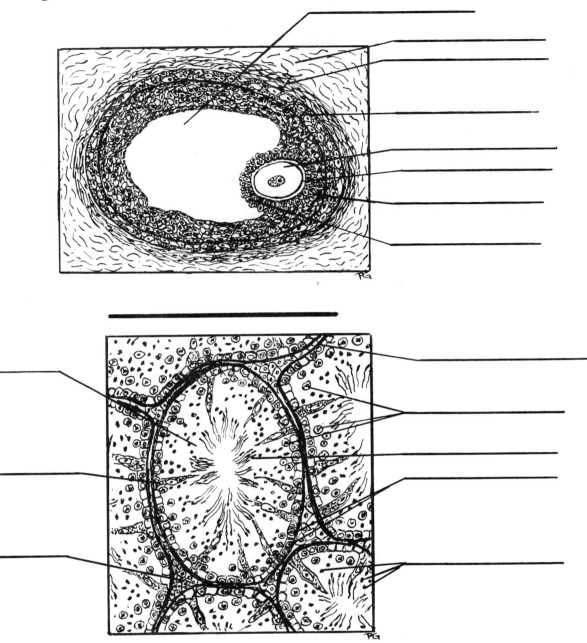

Graafian follicle

antral cavity
corona radiata
cumulus oophorus
membrane granulosa
ovum
theca externa
theca interna
zona pellucida

Testis

basement membrane
interstitial cells (of Leydig)
primary spermatocytes
seminiferous tubule
Sertoli cell
spermatids
spermatogonia
spermatozoa

Slides

Examine the following slides of the reproductive system and make drawings in spaces provided:

1. Testis, c.s.
2. Epididymis, c.s.
3. Prostate gland, c.s.
4. Seminal vesicle, c.s.
5. Ductus deferens, c.s.
6. Sperm smear
7. Ovary, c.s.
8. Corpus luteum, c.s.
9. Oviduct, c.s.
10. Uterus, (cat) resting, c.s.
11. Uterus, (cat) estrus, c.s.
12. Vagina, c.s.

Supply the following labels for each drawing:

1. Testis: tunica albuginea, seminiferous tubule, sertoli cell, spermatocyte, spermatozoa, interstitial cells
2. Epididymis: pseudostratified epithelium, stereocilia (microvilli)
3. Prostate: tubuloalveolar glands, fibroelastic capsule, smooth muscle cells, columnar epithelium, secretion granules
4. Seminal vesicle: mucosa, pseudostratified columnar epithelium, secretion granules
5. Ductus deferens: pseudostratified columnar epithelium, lamina propria, ampulla, smooth muscle cells
6. Sperm smear: head, middle piece, tail
7. Ovary: primordial follicle, Graafian follicle, zona granulosa, antrum, corona radiata, theca interna, theca externa, egg cell
8. Corpus luteum: granulosa lutein cells, theca lutein cells, connective tissue
9. Oviduct: mucosa, columnar epithelium, smooth muscle
10. Uterus: endometrium, myometrium, perimetrium, tubular glands, columnar cells
11. Vagina: stratified squamous epithelium, elastic fibers, lymphocytes, neutrophils, smooth muscle

Draw the following from slides.

Testis (c.s.)

Epididymis (c.s.)

Prostate gland (c.s.)

Seminal vesicle (c.s.)

Ductus deferens (c.s.)

Sperm Smear

Ovary (c.s.)

Corpus luteum (c.s.)

Oviduct (c.s.)

Uterus, (cat) resting, c.s.

Uterus, (cat) estrus, c.s.

Vagina (c.s.)

Questions: Reproductive System

1. The testis is surrounded by a dense fibrous capsule, the _____ _____.

2. The Sertoli cells of the testis are nutritive and are also involved in _____.

3. Leydig (interstitial) cells will secrete _____ after stimulation by the hormone _____.

4. The head portion of a mature spermatozoan will consist of a nucleus and _____.

5. The epididymis is lined with _____ _____ epithelium.

6. The prostate gland is an aggregate of small _____ _____ glands.

7. The layer of cells surrounding the antrum of the follicle and on the outer surface of the zona pellucida is the _____.

8. A follicle after ovulation is known as the _____ _____, which will secrete primarily the hormone _____.

9. The endometrium of the uterus is lined with _____ _____ cells.

10. The lining of the vagina is composed _____ _____ epithelium.

Chapter 15 Endocrine System

The evolution of multicellularity led to the necessity of integrating and coordinating tissues at various and often distant sites in the organism. This need is satisfied by the nervous system and also by the endocrine system. The endocrine system coordinates the various activities of tissues by chemical substances called *hormones,* which are transported by the bloodstream. The tissues and organs that are affected by hormones are called *target organs.* Compared to strictly neural impulses, which are rapid, hormonal stimuli are slower acting, since hormones are stored in the endocrine glands and must be transported by the blood.

The gonads, which are considered endocrine glands in addition to being cytogenic organs, were discussed in the previous sections. The histology of the pituitary (hypophysis), adrenal, thyroid, and parathyroid glands will be discussed in this section.

The Pituitary Gland

The *pituitary gland* is about 1.2 cm × 1.5 cm in size, weighs about 0.5 g, is suspended from the hypothalamus of the brain, and lies in a cavity of the sphenoid bone, the *sella turcica.* It is derived from oral ectoderm (Rathke's pocket) and neural ectoderm (infundibulum or diencephalon). The oral ectoderm gives rise to the *adenohypophysis,* which is composed of the pars distalis (anterior lobe) and pars intermedia (intermediate lobe). The neural ectoderm gives rise to the *neurohypophysis,* which comprises the pars nervosa (posterior lobe) and the infundibulum (neural stalk).

The cells of the anterior lobe are grouped in a typical endocrine gland arrangement in cords and follicles and are classified into two major types, the *chromophobe cells* and the *chromophil cells.* The chromophobe cells are not stained by the usual histological dyes, show few secretory granules under the light microscope, and are smaller than the chromophils. The chromophobes represent undifferentiated precursors of secretory cells or cells in a resting stage. They represent about 50% of the cells of the adenohypophysis.

The chromophil cells contain cytoplasmic granules, are stained by typical dyes, and are subdivided into *acidophils* (35%) and *basophils* (15%) in accordance to their affinity for acidic or basic dyes. The acidophils secrete growth hormone, or somatotropin, (GH, STH) and lactogenic hormone (LTH, prolactin). The basophils secrete adrenocorticotropic hormone (ACTH), thyrotropin (TSH, thyroid-stimulating hormone), follicle-stimulating hormone (FSH), and luteinizing hormone (LH), or interstitial cell-stimulating hormone (ICSH). The hypothalamus of the brain secretes hypophysiotropic hormones (releasing factors), which are transported by the hypophyseal portal circulation to the adenohypophysis. These hypothalamic factors stimulate the cells of the anterior pituitary to release the respective tropic hormones. There are no hypothalamo-adenohyphyseal neural connections.

The cells of the *pars intermedia* (intermediate lobe) are weakly basophilic and are often grouped around vesicles that contain colloid. These cells secrete melanocyte-stimulating hormone (MSH, intermedin), which, in amphibia causes melanocyte dispersal. However, its function in mammals is obscure.

The neurohypophysis of the pituitary consists mainly of unmyelinated axons of secretory nerve cells whose cell bodies are in the supraoptic and paraventricular nuclei of the hypothalamus. The axons terminate blindly in the neural lobe in close relation to capillaries. Small, branching, irregularly shaped cells, the *pituicytes* are observed in the posterior lobe. It is believed that they function primarily as neuroglia, but unlike neuroglia may contain refractile droplets or granules in their cytoplasm, which leads some investigators to believe that they are involved in some secretory function. Neurosecretory granules are observed in the neuron cell body, axon, and in the dilated terminal regions of the axon where they accumulate and are known as *Herring bodies.* Neurosecretion is elaborated in the endoplasmic reticulum (Nissl bodies) of the cell body of the neuron, passing to the Golgi apparatus and along the axons to the hypothalamo-hypophyseal tract to be discharged around the capillaries of the posterior lobe. The supraoptic nuclei are primarily concerned with vasopressin (ADH, antidiuretic hormone) secretion and the paraventricular nuclei are concerned with oxytocin secretion.

The Adrenal Gland

The *adrenal (suprarenal) glands* are paired, somewhat triangular and flattened structures with a combined weight of 10–15 g that are situated in the upper pole of each kidney. Each gland is covered by a capsule of collagenous connective tissue, which surrounds two structurally and functionally distinct regions: the outer adrenal cortex derived from embryonic (coelemic) mesodermal tissues; and the inner adrenal medulla derived from ectodermal neural crest cells. The gland is highly vascular with medullary and cortical arterioles receiving branches from the inferior phrenic, celiac branch of the aorta and the renal artery; venules drain blood to the medullary veins and on to the adrenal veins and vena cava.

Beneath the connective tissue capsule lies the *adrenal cortex,* which consists of an outer zona glomerulosa, followed by a zona fasciculata, zona reticularis, and finally the adrenal medulla.

The cells of the *zona glomerulosa* are columnar, are closely packed and surrounded by capillaries, have a spherical nucleus, a well-developed nucleolus, acidophilic cytoplasm with basophilic granules and lipid droplets, and extensive smooth endoplasmic reticulum, mitochondria, and Golgi apparatus. The cells of the zona glomerulosa secrete the hormone *aldosterone,* a mineral corticoid hormone responsible for potassium excretion and sodium retention (reabsorption) in the distal renal tubule.

The *zona fasciculata* contains polyhedral cells arranged in straight cords one or two cells thick, with the cord running at right angles to the surface of the gland. The cells have a central nucleus, which is occasionally double, slightly basophilic cytoplasm with lipid droplets, microvilli, rough endoplasmic reticulum, and mitochondria. This is the widest zone of the cortex. Adrenocorticotropic hormone (ACTH) from the pituitary stimulates these cells to secrete the hormones cortisone and cortisol (hydrocortisone), which are glucocorticoids responsible for the regulation of carbohydrate, protein, and fat metabolism. Small amounts of estrogens and androgens appear to be produced in the zona fasciculata and in the inner cortical layer, the zona reticularis.

The *zona reticularis* consists of a network of irregular cell cords with cells smaller than those of the fasciculata and with deeply stained nuclei. The cytoplasm is acidophilic with few lipid droplets and it stains darker in routine preparations. Lipofuscin granules are prominent in the cytoplasm. Light and dark forms of these cells have been described but the significance of these forms is not clearly understood. Glucocorticoid hormones such as cortisol and cortisone and possibly sex hormones are secreted by the cells of the zona reticularis.

The *adrenal medulla* is composed of round or polyhedral cells arranged in clumps or short cords and surrounded by capillaries and a few sympathetic ganglion cells. The cells stain light purple in H&E preparations and are basophilic. When oxidizing agents such as chromate are used, the cells stain brown and are therefore called chromaffin cells. Based on differences of the structure of cell granules and on histochemical studies, two cell types have been identified. One with medium electron density granules secreting the catecholamine epinephrine and the other with intense electron density granule secreting norepinephrine. Secretion of these hormones is under the direct control of the sympathetic nervous system. Epinephrine increases cardiac output, elevates blood glucose, and increases the basal metabolic rate. Norepinephrine acts primarily to elevate blood pressure by vasoconstriction of peripheral capillaries.

The Thyroid Gland

The *thyroid gland* is located ventral to the larynx, weighs 30 – 40 g, and consists of two lateral lobes separated by an isthmus. A loose connective tissue capsule of reticular fibers covers the gland and sends septa into the gland separating the spherical follicles. The follicles are composed of a single layer of cuboidal epithelium resting on a basement membrane. The nuclei are spherical, occupy a central position, and contain one or more nucleoli. Mitochondria are evenly distributed in the cytoplasm. The epithelium surrounds a central gelatinous colloid. There is an extensive vascular network. The gland is innervated by the sympathetic and parasympathetic nervous system. The height of the cells of the thyroid epithelium is related to the functional activity of the gland. In a gland involved in average secretory activity, the epithelium is cuboidal. Inactive cells are squamous, whereas hyperactive cells are columnar and tend to fill up the central cavity by squeezing the colloid. Golgi and microvilli are seen in the apical region of the cell. A granular endoplasmic reticulum is at the basal region and mitochondria are dispersed throughout the cytoplasm.

The synthesis of thyroid hormone by the epithelial cells is controlled by pituitary TSH, which in turn is affected by hypothalamic releasing factors. The synthesis of thyroid hormone takes place as follows:

1. Amino acids enter the basal portion of the cell and are synthesized to polypeptides with the incorporation of a carbohydrate moiety into a noniodinate glyco-protein, thyroglobulin, which enters the colloid.
2. Iodide is taken up by the follicle cells and oxidized by peroxidase to iodine. The iodine reaches the thyroglobulin in the colloid where it unites with the tyrosine groups in the molecule to iodinate the thyroglobulin and to form

monoiodotyrosine (MIT) and dioiodotyrosine (DIT) with eventual coupling to give rise to triiodothyronine (T3) and tetraiodothyronine (T4) (thyroxin).

3. Iodinated thyroglobulin containing T3 and T4 is reabsorbed at the region of the microvilli by pinocytosis. Enzymes from lysosomes liberate into the cytoplasm MIT, DIT, T3, and T4 from the thyroglobulin. The T3 and T4 cross the basal region of the cell and enter the capillaries, are bound to plasma proteins, and circulate to affect target organs. The thyroid hormones (T3 and T4) affect calorigenesis, body growth, carbohydrate absorption, and lipid metabolism.

Parathyroid Glands

The *parathyroid glands* are small paired glands, usually four in number, which lie on the posterior surface of the thyroid gland. Each parathyroid gland is contained within a connective tissue capsule, which sends septa to the inside of the gland. The parenchyma consists of two types of cells:

1. *chief cells* (principal cells), which measure 7–10 μm in diameter are most numerous, polygonal with a vesicular nucleus and a slightly acidophilic cytoplasm with granules [probably containing parathyroid hormone (PTH)], prominent Golgi, rough (granular) endoplasmic reticulum (rER), spherical mitochondria, and lipofuscin pigment bodies.
2. *oxyphil cells,* which are larger than chief cells and polygonal in shape, with acidophilic granules in the cytoplasm, which are mitochondria.

Parathyroid hormone (PTH) secreted by the chief cells controls the level of calcium and phosphate ions in the blood. A decrease in blood calcium stimulates the secretion of PTH, which acts on the osteoclast cells of the bone to cause cell resorption and subsequent calcium release into the blood. Conversely, PTH reduces the level of phosphate in the blood by increasing phosphate excretion in the kidney.

The effects of PTH are reversed by the hormone thyrocalcitonin. This hormone lowers the blood calcium levels, stimulates osteoblast activity, and increases blood phosphate. This hormone is secreted by the parafollicular cells (C-shaped, clear, or light cells), which lie adjacent to the thyroid follicles. These cells are larger than follicular cells and have eccentric nuclei and numerous membrane-bound, dense cytoplasmic granules.

Pituitary

Label illustrations using terms below.

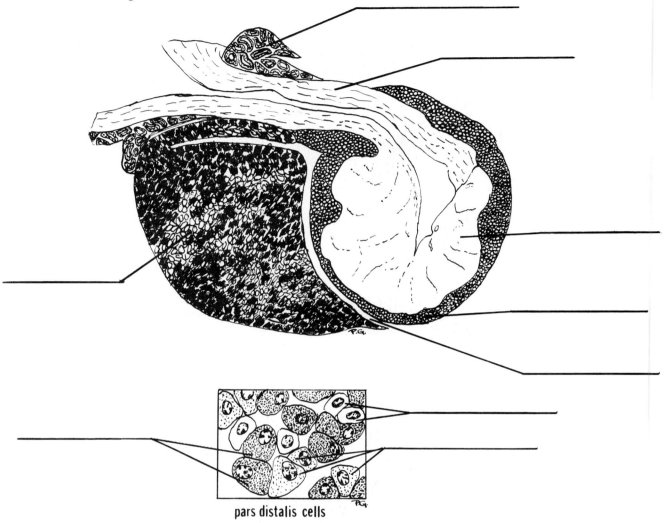

pars distalis cells

cleft
infundibular stalk (containing nerve tracts)
pars distalis (anterior lobe)
acidophils
basophils
chromophobes
pars intermedia
pars nervosa (posterior lobe)

Adrenal Gland, Parathyroid, and Thyroid

Label illustrations using terms listed below.

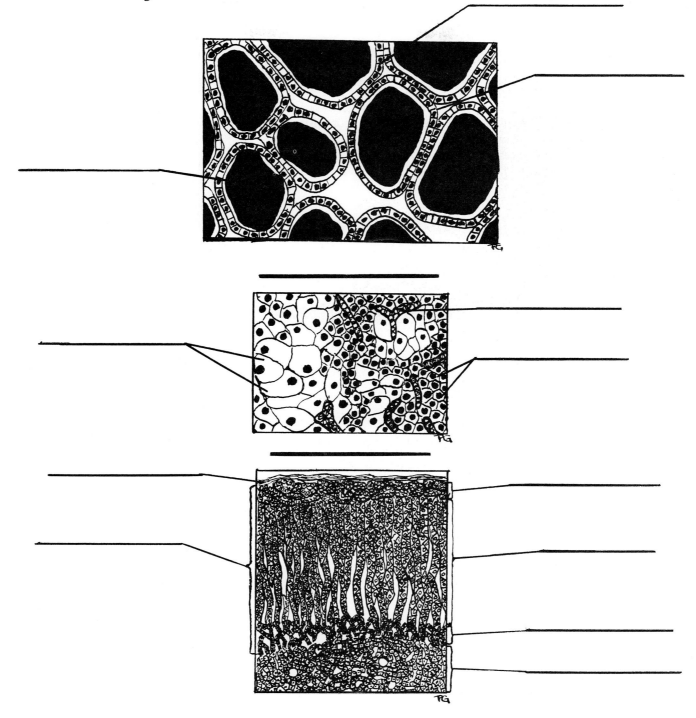

Adrenal gland
cortex
zona glomerulosa
zona fasciculata
zona reticularis
medulla

Parathyroid
capillary
chief cells
oxyphil cells

Thyroid
colloid
cuboidal (epithelium)
follicle

Slides

Examine the following slides of the endocrine system and make drawings in spaces provided:

1. Pituitary gland, l.s.
2. Adrenal gland, c.s.
3. Thyroid gland, c.s.
4. Parathyroid gland, c.s.

Supply the following labels for each drawing:

1. Pituitary gland: pars distalis, pars intermedia, pars nervosa, acidophils, basophils, chromophobes, pituicytes
2. Adrenal gland: zona glomerulosa, zona fasciculata, zona reticularis, medulla
3. Thyroid gland: follicle, cuboidal epithelium, colloid, parafollicular cells
4. Parathyroid gland: chief cells, oxyphil cells

Draw the following from slides.

Pituitary gland—anterior (l.s.)

Pituitary glan—posterior (l.s.)

Adrenal gland (c.s.)

Thyroid gland (c.s.)

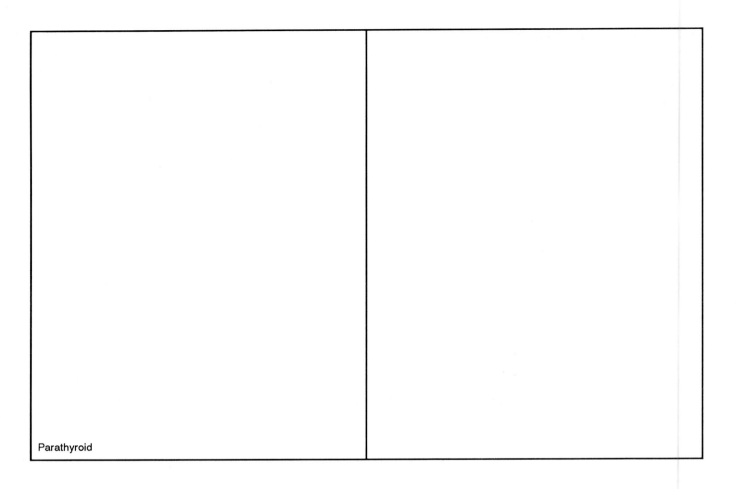

Parathyroid

Questions: Endocrine System

1. The embryological origin of the pituitary anterior lobe is _____, whereas the posterior lobe is derived from _____.

2. Anterior lobe chromophil cells are subdivided, according to staining reactions, into _____ and _____.

3. Hypothalamic hormones will be transported to the adenohypophysis by the _____ circulation.

4. Neurosecretory granules in the neurohypophysis are known as _____ _____.

5. The hypothalamic supraoptic nuclei are primarily concerned with the secretion of the posterior lobe hormone _____.

6. The embryological origin of the adrenal cortex is _____, whereas the adrenal medulla is derived from _____.

7. Located beneath the capsule of the adrenal cortex is the histological layer _____ _____ whose cells secrete the hormone _____.

8. Cortisone and cortisol are secreted by the cells of the _____ _____ layer of the cortex.

9. Thyroid follicles are composed of _____ epithelium.

10. The chief cells of the parathyroid secrete the hormone _____ whereas the thyroid parafollicular cells secrete the hormone _____.

Histological Microtechnique

Introduction

Histological microtechniques are often included in laboratory courses on histology. Familiarity with the basic principles and procedures of tissue fixation, sectioning, and differential staining should lead to a deeper understanding of tissue structure and function. Many tissues, cells, and cell components are identified and even classified according to their affinity to specific stains. Examples of such cells are neutrophils, acidophils, eosinophils, basophils, argyrophils, chromophils, and chromophobes.

The development of magnifying lenses and simple microscopes preceded the refinement of techniques used in the preservation and preparation of cells and tissues for detailed study. Magnifying lenses were used by the Romans. Spectacled lenses of molded and polished glass were used in the thirteenth century. Janssens in Holland is credited with the invention of the microscope in 1590. Improvements in microscopy were subsequently made in the seventeenth century by Borelli, Malpighi, Hooke, and van Leeuwenhoek. However, it was not until the development of compound lenses and substage condensers in the later part of the nineteenth century that microscopy reached a level of improvement approaching modern standards.

Practical techniques in fixation, sectioning, and staining were developed late in the nineteenth century. These developments occurred about two hundred years after the microscope improvements of the seventeenth century. A table model microtome with a slanting top was used by His in 1866. Rotary microtomes were developed by Pfeifer (1883), Minot (1886), and Spencer (1910). Sliding microtomes were developed by Bausch and Lomb Optical (1882). However, ultramicrotomes for thin sections used in electron microscopy were not developed until 1956 by Richards. Paraffin embedding procedures were developed by Klebs (1869) and Butchli (1881).

Natural dyes and stains, such as the invaluable Tyrian purple (royal purple) extracted from a gastropod mollusc, have been known since ancient times. Acetocarmine, which is used for chromosome staining, is extracted from a homopteran insect and was first used by Belling in 1921. Hematoxylin, one of the most important histological stains first used about 1863, is extracted from a Central and South American logwood tree related to the acacia tree. Other natural dyes are saffron (from the stigmas of crocus), indigo (blue-violet from the tropical shrub indigofera), berberine (yellow crystal from the bark of barberry), and brazilin (red from brazilwood Caesalpina).

Synthetic dyes and stains were first developed by the German chemical industry in the late nineteenth century and were first used on biological materials by Paul Ehrlich (1896). This led to Ehrlich's concept of specific staining and selective toxicity, which was followed by his early discovery of a treatment for syphilis. Ehrlich is considered the father of chemotherapy. The use of selective stains in chemotherapy also led to the discovery of the sulfa drugs by Domagk in 1936. Commonly used synthetic stains in microtechnique include aceto-orcein (red) used for chromosomal staining, eosin Y (orange) as a cytoplasmic counterstain, fast green FCF (green) as a counterstain and Wright stain for blood.

Preparation of Tissues

Preparation of tissues includes (1) fixation, (2) dehydration, (3) clearing, (4) infiltration, (5) embedding, (6) sectioning, and (7) staining.

Fixation

Living and unstained cells and tissues may be studied by phase contrast microscopy. However, unless living cells and tissues are maintained under conditions of cell culture, they deteriorate rapidly and permanency cannot be maintained for future reference. Many structures are ill defined under such conditions and can only be clearly differentiated by the use of stains. Relatively nontoxic dyes such as trypan blue or neutral red, which do not kill cells or tissues, may be used as vital stains. Since most stains kill the tissues, it is necessary to appropriately prepare tissues by fixation, dehydration, clearing, infiltration, embedding, and sectioning before staining. These procedures must be applied selectively according to the tissues utilized, in order to prevent tissue distortion and artifact formation. Various tissues because of their diverse composition generally require different fixatives.

Fixation renders the structural components of cells insoluble by the precipitation of the proteins and other classes of compounds. Tissues should be placed in fixatives as soon as possible after dissection in order to prevent bacterial putrefaction and autolysis by lysosomal enzymes. If autolysis begins to take place, amino acids will diffuse out of the cells and cell proteins can no longer be coagulated by chemical agents such as fixatives. Such cell changes are called *post mortem* conditions.

Objectives of tissue preparation are (1) to prevent post mortem changes, (2) to differentiate the solid phase of cell components from the aqueous phase, (3) to alter cell structures into materials that will remain insoluble during subsequent treatment, (4) to protect cells from distortion and shrinkage when subjected to alcohols and hot paraffin, (5) to improve the staining potential, (6) to improve the refractive index of tissues for better visibility.

Requirements of a fixative are (1) rapid penetration of tissues, (2) coagulation of soluble cell components, (3) protection of tissues against shrinkage and distortion during dehydration, embedding, and sectioning, (4) improvement of staining potential and enhancement of the distinguishing cell structures.

The choice of a fixative should be determined by the purpose for which the tissue is to be stained or preserved. Solutions of a single chemical seldom have all of the properties of a good fixative. Mixtures are usually employed since different components have different actions. The choice of a fixative will depend upon the properties of the tissue and the subsequent stain to be used. To ensure rapid penetration, tissue blocks should be less than 4 mm thick and should be immersed in fixative at least ten times their volume.

Proteins fixatives are classified as coagulating fixatives and denaturing fixatives.

Coagulating fixatives cause a coarse polymerization of protein molecules resulting in the formation of a precipitate similar to the effect of thermocoagulation. Examples of coagulating fixatives are methanol, ethanol, nitric acid, trichloroacetic acid, mercuric chloride, picric acid, and chromic acid. These fixatives are found in solutions of Gilson, Heidenhain, Zenker, Carnoy, Flemming, and Bouin.

Denaturing (noncoagulating) *fixatives* render the proteins insoluble by internal rearrangement, cross-linking, and fixative binding without forming precipitates. These fixatives are suited to fine cytological and histochemical procedures and some are also commonly used in electron microscopy. Examples of denaturing fixatives are osmium tetroxide, potassium dichromate, acetic acid, formalin, and glutaraldehyde. These fixatives are found in solutions of Zenker-formalin (Helly), Flemming, Champey, Hermann, and Bouin. Ten percent buffered neutral formalin may be used alone and is compatible with most stains.

Dehydration

For paraffin infiltration and embedding, tissues must be dehydrated and cleared in solutions miscible with paraffin since paraffin is not miscible in water. Dehydration is the removal of all extractable water by dehydrants such as ethanol (most widely used), isopropanol (causes minimal shrinkage but most dyes are not soluble in its solution), butyl alcohol (miscible in paraffin but disagreeable odor), and Solox (denatures ethanol and methanol). In order to prevent shrinkage, in transferring tissues from lower to higher concentrations, dehydration must be gradual.

Clearing

Clearing is an intermediate step following dehydration and preceding paraffin infiltration. Clearing agents must be miscible with the dehydrant and paraffin. The clearing agent clears the opacity from the dehydrated tissues making them translucent. Xylene is the most widely used clearing agent and has fast action but tends to harden tissues if they are immersed in its solution for more than one hour. Other clearing agents are benzene (high evaporation, less hardening, overnight action), toluene (less hardening, overnight action), chloroform (highly volatile), methyl benzoate (nonhardening, overnight action), and dioxane (miscible in water and paraffin, fast acting, slight shrinkage, very toxic).

Infiltration

Infiltration is the complete removal of the clearing agent by the substitution of melted paraffin. Paraffin and paraffin preparations of various melting points are available such as Paraplast (containing paraffin and plastic polymers and available as "soft paraffin" with melting points of 50–52°C or 53–55°C or as "hard paraffin" with melting points of 56–58°C or 60–68°C). Other paraffins or paraffin preparations are pure paraffin (not generally used—sections compress and wrinkle), paraffin plus beeswax (generally satisfactory), Tissuemat (commercial preparation of paraffin and additives, generally equivalent to Paraplast), Bioloid paraffin (commercial mixture of paraffin and other waxes). Choice of paraffin

use-hard paraffin, cold weather use-soft paraffin). Generally, paraffin with the most useful melting point is one with a melting point of 56–58°C.

Embedding

Embedding is the orientation of tissue in melted paraffin, which when solidified provides a firm medium for the tissue and enables sectioning without tissue damage or distortion. Melted paraffin must be fully molten to properly infiltrate but its temperature must not be higher than just enough to maintain it in the molten state. Most tissues should not be left in molten paraffin more than a total of four hours, otherwise tissue hardening and shrinkage may result. Tissues in a hardened paraffin block may be stored indefinitely.

Sectioning

The hardened paraffin block containing the tissue should be mounted on a microtome carrier and trimmed with a blade in a square or parallel shape. Square corners are essential in order to get a straight ribbon when sectioning. For typical tissues such as liver or duodenum sections should be made at 10 m. Glass slides cleaned in laboratory detergent, dipped in 95% ethanol, and air dried should be available. Slides should be coated lightly with Mayer's albumen adhesive fixative and covered with a slight film of water upon which the paraffin ribbon will be floated. The slide with the floating ribbon should then be placed on a hot plate adjusted to 45°C until the water evaporates and the ribbon has adhered to the glass slide. Some technicians float the ribbon on a warmed water bath to straighten out the ribbon and then place it in a slide. The slide is now ready to be immersed in a clearing agent for paraffin removal and subsequent hydration and staining.

Staining

Most stains in histology are acid or base stains, however, they are not acids or bases per se, but neutral salts that dissolve into anions (–)(acid radicals) or cations (+)(basic radicals). The component that imparts color is in the anion or cation of the dissociated salt. For example, hematoxylin is a basic or cationic stain that will stain acidic structures such as nuclear elements. Conversely, eosin is an acid or anionic stain that will stain basic cytoplasmic components.

Certain stains such as hematoxylin require a *mordant* to form a base for the dye, which will then stain acidic nuclear components. A mordant is a metallic salt or hydroxide that combines with a dye radical to form an insoluble compound called a "lake." The mordant-dye compound is relatively permanent and is insoluble in neutral solutions. It can be followed by other methods of staining. Typical mordants are aluminum, ferric and chromium salts, potassium, ammonium, iron and chrome alum, and ferric chloride. In preparing hematoxylin stains, the crystals of hematoxylin are not a dye until the color is allowed to "develop" or "ripen" by oxidation into hematein. Types of hematoxylin are

1. Delafield–six weeks to ripen, keeps indefinitely
2. Ehrlich–six to eight weeks to ripen, keeps indefinitely
3. Harris–immediate, but does not keep longer than one to two months
4. Heidenhain's iron hematoxylin–immediate upon mixing solutions 1 and 2, keeps up to three months

Examples of basic stains that stain nuclei, basophilic granules, and some bacteria are alcian blue, azure A & C, basic fuschin, carmine, hematoxylin, Janus green B, methyl green, methylene blue, neutral red, orcein, safranine O, and toluidine blue. Examples of acid stains that stain cytoplasm, acidophilic granules, and basic tissue components are acid fuschin, aniline blue, congo red, eosin, fast green, orange G, and phloxine B.

Procedures

The following organs should be dissected from a mouse or rat, rinsed in physiological saline, and cut to appropriate size for fixation and subsequent preparation: liver (lv), duodenum (du), heart (ht), esophagus (es), pancreas (pa), kidney (kd), testis (ts), and ovary (ov).

A. Fixation
   1. Bouin's fixative
      a. Fix tissues 12 to 24 hours (storage for several weeks causes no damage).
      b. Wash in running water (1 hr); transfer to 50% alcohol (ethanol) (1/2 hr); transfer to 70% alcohol with a few drops of saturated lithium carbonate (1/2 hr) or until yellow color disappears; tissues may be stored indefinitely in 70% alcohol.

b. Wash in running water (1 hr); transfer to 50% alcohol (ethanol) (1/2 hr); transfer to 70% alcohol with a few drops of saturated lithium carbonate (1/2 hr) or until yellow color disappears; tissues may be stored indefinitely in 70% alcohol.

2. Carnoy's fixative
   a. Fix tissues twenty minutes to three hours depending on the size of the tissue.
   b. Transfer to 95% alcohol (1 hr); then to 70% alcohol (for temporary storage if necessary) or dehydrate immediately.

B. Dehydration
A requirement for paraffin sectioning is proper infiltration and embedding, which must have been preceded by dehydration. Fixed tissues should be transferred from 70% alcohol to 95% alcohol (1/2 hr); 100% absolute alcohol (1/2 hr); second 100% absolute alcohol (1 hr).

C. Clearing
Transfer dehydrated tissues as follows: 1 xylene-1 absolute alcohol (15 min); xylene I (15 min); xylene II (15 min); xylene-saturated paraffin (15 min at 35°C).

D. Infiltration
Transfer cleared tissues in paraffin oven at 56–58°C as follows: paraffin I (30 min); paraffin II (30 min); paraffin III (1 hr).

E. Embedding
Pour melted (fresh) paraffin into tissue capsule; transfer and orient tissue in melted paraffin; allow tissue capsule to cool until film appears on the surface and then immerse tissue capsule in cold water. The block in the tissue capsule can now be mounted on a microtome for sectioning.

F. Sectioning
Sectioning in a typical course in histology and histological technique is usually done with a standard rotary microtome. The techniques of proper sectioning can best be demonstrated by a laboratory instructor.

Stains

Hematoxylin and Eosin (Delafield's hematoxylin and eosin Y)

After fixation (any general fixative), dehydration, clearing, infiltration, embedding, and sectioning, transfer the slides through the following solutions:

1. xylene I, 5 min
2. xylene II, 2 min
3. 100% alcohol, 2 min
4. 95% alcohol, 2 min
5. 70% alcohol, 2 min (with saturated lithium carbonate following Bouin's fixative)
6. 50% alcohol, 2 min
7. 35% alcohol, 2 min
8. water, 2 min
9. Delafield's hematoxylin, 3–5 min
10. rinse in running water and check slide under a microscope for understaining or overstaining
11. 35% alcohol, 2 min
12. 50% alcohol, 2 min
13. 70% alcohol, 2 min [if overstained, transfer into acid/alcohol (two drops concentrated HCl in 70% alcohol) until sections are red-purple]
14. 95% alcohol, 2 min
15. eosin Y solution (0.5 g, eosin Y in 100 ml 95% ethanol, 2–5 min)
16. 95% alcohol, 2–3 min. to rinse off excess eosin
17. 100% alcohol, 2 min
18. 100% alcohol, 2 min
19. xylene, 2 min
20. xylene, 2 min
21. mount slide with cover slip using mounting medium such as Permount

Results—blue: nuclei; orange: cytoplasm, connective tissue fibers, muscle fibrils

Methylene Blue-phloxine

After fixation (any general fixative), dehydration, clearing, infiltration, embedding, and sectioning, transfer the slides through the following solutions:

1. xylene I, 5 min
2. xylene II, 2 min
3. 100% alcohol, 2 min
4. 95% alcohol, 2 min
5. 70% alcohol, 2 min (with saturated lithium carbonate following Bouin's fixative)
6. 50% alcohol, 2 min
7. 35% alcohol, 2 min
8. water, 2 min
9. phloxine solution, 1 min (phloxine 0.5 g, water 100 ml, glacial acetic acid 0.2 ml)
10. rinse in water
11. methylene blue solution, 1 min (methylene blue 0.25 g, azure B 0.25 g, borax 0.25 g, water 100 ml)
12. wash excess blue quickly in 0.2% aqueous acetic acid
13. 95% alcohol, rinse 1 min
14. 95% alcohol, rinse 1 min
15. 95% alcohol, rinse 1 min
16. 100% alcohol, 2 min
17. 100% alcohol, 2 min
18. xylene, 2 min
19. xylene, 2 min
20. mount slide with cover slip using mounting medium such as Permount

Results—blue: nuclei, cytoplasmic basophils, goblet cell mucin; pink: cytoplasm, collagen, muscle fibrils

Feulgen Method for DNA

Feulgen in 1924 first used the Schiff reaction on aldehydes to stain DNA. Hydrolysis with HCl will liberate the aldehyde groups from the deoxypentose sugars of DNA. The aldehydes will react with Schiff reagent to give a red-violet (magenta) color.

After fixation (Carnoy's fixative preferred; Bouin's not recommended), dehydration, clearing, infiltration, embedding, and sectioning, transfer the slides through the following solutions:

1. xylene I, 5 min
2. xylene II, 2 min
3. 100% alcohol, 2 min
4. 95% alcohol, 2 min
5. 70% alcohol, 2 min
6. 50% alcohol, 2 min
7. 35% alcohol, 2 min
8. water, 2 min
9. hydrolyze in 1 N HCl at 60°C for 6 min
10. water, 30 sec
11. Schiff reagent, 2 hrs (in the dark)
12. bleaching solution (rinse three times at 2 min each) (5 ml 1 N HCl, 5 ml 10% aqueous sodium metabisulfite, 100 ml water)
13. water, 1 min
14. fast green FCF, 8 sec (0.05 g fast green, 100 ml 95% alcohol)
15. rinse in 95% alcohol
16. 100% alcohol, 2 min
17. 100% alcohol, 2 min
18. xylene, 2 min
19. xylene, 2 min
20. mount slide with cover slip using mounting medium such as Permount

Results—red: DNA (chromosomes); green: cytoplasm, nucleoli

Periodic Acid-Schiff (PAS) Method for Glycogen

Carbohydrates will yield aldehyde groups when oxidized by periodic acid. The aldehyde groups will react with Schiff reagent to give a red-violet color. This staining reaction is excellent in demonstrating glycogen in goblet cells of the digestive tract.

After fixation (Carnoy's fixative preferred), dehydration, clearing, infiltration, embedding, and sectioning, transfer the slides through the following solutions:

1. xylene I, 5 min
2. xylene II, 2 min
3. 100% alcohol, 2 min
4. 95% alcohol, 2 min
5. 70% alcohol, 2 min
6. 50% alcohol, 2 min
7. 35% alcohol, 2 min
8. water, 2 min
9. periodic acid, 5 min (1 g periodic acid, 100 ml water)
10. rinse in running tap water, 5 min
11. Schiff reagent, 10 min
12. sulfite rinse, three times at 2 min each (0.5 g sodium metabisulfite, 100 ml water)
13. rinse in running tap water, 5 min
14. Delafield's hematoxylin (counterstain), 2 min
15. rinse in running tap water until section is blue
16. 35% alcohol, 2 min
17. 50% alcohol, 2 min
18. 70% alcohol, 2 min
19. 95% alcohol, 2 min
20. 100% alcohol, 2 min
21. 100% alcohol, 2 min
22. xylene, 2 min
23. xylene, 2 min
24. mount slide with cover slip using mounting medium such as Permount

Results—red: glycogen, cartilage, mucin, starch; blue: nucleus

Index

loose connective tissue, 27
LTH, 145
luteal phase, 137
luteinizing hormone, 137
lymph, 48
lymphatic tissue, 28
lymphocytes, 51
lymphoid cells, 118

M-line, 64
macrocytes, 48
macrophage, 27, 30, 119
macula densa, 126
male reproductive system, 135
Malpighian pyramids, 125
mast cells, 27, 31
maturation division, 135
mature follicle, 137
Mazia, Daniel, 1
mediastinum testis, 135
medium sized arteries, 84
medium sized veins, 84
medulla-hair, 93
medullary pyramids, 125
medullary rays, 125
medullary region of ovary, 137
megakaryocytes, 51
meiosis, 135
Meissner's plexus, 100
melanin, 92
melanoblasts, 92
melanocytes, 92
membraneous urethra, 126
menstrual cycle, phase, 138
merocrine, 93
mesenchymal epithelial, 18
mesenchyme, 48
mesoderm, 15
mesothelium, 18
metaphase I and II, 135
metarterioles, 83
microcytes, 48
microfibrils, 28
microglia, 75
microtubules-nervous, 72
middle disc, 64
middle piece, 136
mitochondrial sheath, 136
Mittelscheibe, 64
mixed gland, 109
monocytes, 51
motor end plate, 73
motor unit, 73
MSH, 145
mucigen, 18
mucin, 18
mucopolysaccharide, 18
mucosa, 99
mucosal pit, 100
mucous cells, 109
mucous neck cells, 100
Müllerian duct, 126
multipolar neuron, 72
muscle, 64
muscle spindle, 73
muscular arteries, 82, 84
muscular layer, 110
muscularis mucosae, 99
myelin sheath, 72
myeloblast, 57

myelocytes, 57
myeloid tissue, 28
myelopoiesis, 57
myoblast, 66
myocardium, 85
myoepithelial cells, 93
myofibrils, 64
myofilaments, 64
myoid cells, 135
myometrium, 137
myosin, 64

nasopharynx, 118
neck-sperm, 136
nephrons, 125
nerve fibers, 73
nerve trunk, 72
nervous system, 72
neural stalk, 145
neurofibrils, 72
neurofilaments, 72
neuroglia, 72, 75
neurons, 72
neuroplasm, 72
neutrophilic myelocytes, 57
neutrophils, 48
Nissl bodies, 72
nodes of Ranvier, 73
non-encapsulated nerve endings, 73
non-granular leucocytes, 51
non-keratinized squamous epithelium, 118
normoblasts, 57
notochord, 27
nutritive cells, 135

olfactory cells, 118
olfactory epithelium, 118
olfactory region, 118
oligodendria, 75
oocyte, 137
osteoblasts, 40
osteoclasts, 40
osteocytes, 40
osteone, 40
outer epithelial root sheath, 93
outer fibrous layer, 40
outer main gland, 136
outer papillary, 92
ovaries, 137
oviduct, 137
Owen, Richard, 1
oxyphil cells, 147
oxytocin, 145

pachytene, 135
Pacinian corpuscles, 73
paired dorsal artery, 136
pancreas, 99, 109
papillary ducts of Bellini, 126
parafollicular cells, 147
paralutein cells, 137
parasympathetic stimulation, 136
parathyroid gland, 147
parathyroid hormone, 147
paraventricular nuclei, 145
parenchyma, 109
parietal cells, 100
parietal layer, 125
parotid gland, 109
pars distalis, 145

pars intermedia, 145
pars nervosa, 145
pedicels, 125
penis, 126
pepsin, 100
pericardium, 85
perichondrium, 39
perikaryon, 72
perimetrium, 137
perimysium, 66
perineurium, 72
perineuronal, 75
periosteum, 40
peripheral glands, 93
perivascular, 75
Peyer's patches, 30, 100
pigment, 92
pituicytes, 145
pituitary anterior lobe, 145
pituitary gland, 145
pituitary intermediate lobe, 145
pituitary posterior lobe, 145
plasma cells, 27, 31
podocytes, 125
polychromatic erythroblasts, 57
portal canals, 109
portal vein, 109
postganglionic visceral fibers, 73
pre-cartilage, 27
precapillary arterioles, 83
precapillary sphincters, 82
premenstrual phase, 138
prickle cells, 92
primary bronchi, 118
primary oocyte, 137
primary spermatocytes, 135
primordial follicle, 137
principal piece, 136
proerythroblast cells, 57
prolactin, 145
proliferative phase, 138
promyeloblasts, 57
prophase I and II, 135
prostate gland, 126
prostatic urethra, 126
prostatic utricle, 126
prothrombin, 53
protoplasm, 1
protoplasmic astrocyte, 75
proximal centriole, 136
proximal convoluted tubule, 125
pseudostratified epithelial, 18
PTH, 147
Purkinje, 1
Purkinje fibers, 86
pyloric gland, 100

Rathke's pocket, 145
RBC, 48
relaxin, 41
renal capsule, 125
renal corpuscle, 125
renal cortex, 125
renal medulla, 125
renal papillae, 125
renal pelvis, 125
renin, 125
respiratory system, 118
rete testis, 136
reticular fibers, 27, 28